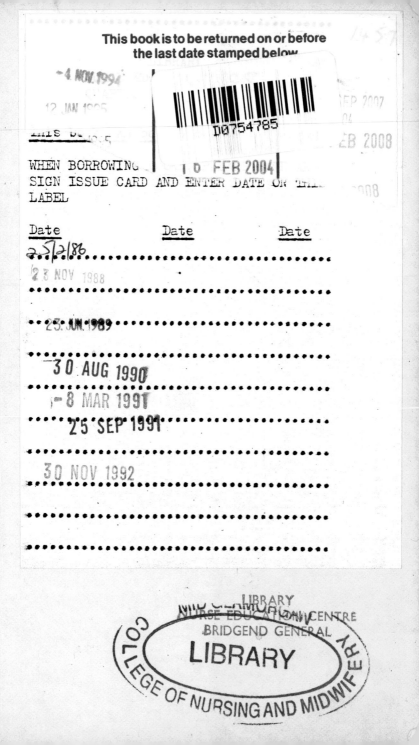

Living with Multiple Sclerosis

By the same author

ASTHMA, HAY FEVER AND OTHER ALLERGIES,
AND HOW TO LIVE WITH THEM
(*William Luscombe Publisher Limited*)

Living with Multiple Sclerosis

ELIZABETH FORSYTHE
M.R.C.S., L.R.C.P., D.P.H.

FABER AND FABER
London & Boston

First published in 1979
by Faber and Faber Limited
3 Queen Square London WC1N 3AU
Reprinted 1980
Printed in Great Britain by
Redwood Burn Limited
Trowbridge & Esher
All rights reserved

© *Elizabeth Forsythe, 1979*

British Library Cataloguing in Publication Data

Forsythe, Elizabeth
Living with multiple sclerosis.
1. Multiple sclerosis
I. Title
616.8'34   RC277

ISBN 0–571–11293–5
ISBN 0–571–11294–3   Pbk

Change of address: see pages 126 and 137

The Multiple Sclerosis Society
286 Munster Road, London SW6 6AP
Telephone 01-381 4022

Contents

ONE	Diagnosis and Before	*page* 7
TWO	Multiple Sclerosis as a Disease	15
THREE	Some Medical and Patient Mythology	25
FOUR	Acceptance	33
FIVE	Adjustments	40
SIX	Early Treatment	47
SEVEN	Multiple Sclerosis and Diet	53
EIGHT	Exercise and Rest	62
NINE	Friends and Help	69
TEN	Getting Through the Bad Patches	75
ELEVEN	Multiple Sclerosis and the Family	82
TWELVE	Multiple Sclerosis and its Mental Effects	89
THIRTEEN	Multiple Sclerosis and Work	95
FOURTEEN	Doctors	101
FIFTEEN	Identity as Able or Disabled	108
SIXTEEN	Sources of Information	115
SEVENTEEN	Statutory Services	121
EIGHTEEN	The Voluntary Societies	126
NINETEEN	Facing the Future	132
	Useful Books	136
	Useful Addresses	137
	Useful Information Relating to the U.S.A.	138
	Index	139

CHAPTER ONE

Diagnosis and Before

Mine is a common story and happens in different ways to many people each year. Now that the incidents have become part of my life I can look back on the past two years with neither surprise nor horror, nor any feeling of bitterness.

I was born, brought up, and educated in the south of England and spent my teenage years there during the Second World War. I qualified as a doctor in a London medical school and worked for a time in London before going into country general practice. Looking back now, with the benefit of hindsight, I can remember that I had a mysteriously weak left leg, which started at the end of my final examinations. I do remember that there were some neurological signs in the leg and it was thought that there might be pressure on a nerve in my back. It cleared up after many weeks of rest. Following that incident I had periods of extreme fatigue while doing my early resident jobs. Of course, we all got tired because we worked about eighteen hours a day and were frequently called at night. It now seems to me that the fatigue was excessive because during my student days I had been remarkably healthy and managed to combine a very hectic social life, a lot of interests and enough hard work to do well in examinations. After the weak leg I never had the same resilience again. At times the fatigue was so extreme that I had to stop working for a while. It was never considered that I could have a physical illness but was probably attributed to 'neurasthenia' or possibly in more basic language —lack of guts.

I had wanted to specialise in children's medicine and during my student days was encouraged in this ambition by those for whom I worked. There seemed no doubt that I should have the physical and mental ability to take higher examinations. This attitude changed after I qualified and I started to have periods of fatigue. Not only did I lose confidence in my own ability to succeed but I lost the support of those senior to me on whose help my future would, to a large extent, have depended. It became clear that I lacked the necessary capacity for hard work to succeed in a competitive profession.

At the time I was bitterly disappointed and very depressed at what seemed to me to be failure through my own lack of will power. Rather than potter along in the world of hospital medicine with little hope of success, I decided to abandon all my former ambitions and work as an assistant in rural general practice. I was very fortunate with the practice in which I started training near Cambridge. I found my colleagues congenial and helpful and I found that I could manage the work without undue fatigue. I forgot about my disappointment and frustration and threw myself wholeheartedly into this new world of country practice. Life seemed good again; I could manage the work and found it interesting and my morale was restored. I more or less forgot about my previous patches of ill health but some lack of confidence in my health probably remained.

I married and we had three children. At the time I should have said that everything went very well with the pregnancies but again with hindsight I can remember that I had a spell of double vision after the birth of the second child. I saw an oculist who said that it was probably due to fatigue and that I should get as much rest as possible. Life at the time was fairly hectic because the two children were born twenty months apart. There was little time for reading or sewing so that I was not unduly troubled by the double vision and I think it cleared up in about three months. Before and after the birth of the third child I had a weak left hand and a feeling of heaviness in both lower legs. It was hot weather and as I had two other small children to look after, again it seemed quite reasonable to put it down to fatigue. Eventually some months after the birth these problems cleared up.

Some twelve years ago we bought land and ruins in the north

of Scotland in the area from where my husband's forbears had come. We had at first intended to convert some old crofts into a holiday home; my husband, being considerably older than I, was already beginning to think about retirement and in 1969 I suggested that we should make the ruined crofts a permanent home when he retired. He thought it was a marvellous idea but was doubtful whether I, who had spent all my life in the south of England, would be happy to settle there! We investigated the possibility of schools for the children. They were all at private schools in the south but the increasing cost of private secondary schooling had been looming, and especially in view of my husband's retirement, we both believed they might fare better with a State secondary education in Scotland rather than in England. The local high school in Scotland seemed to be more than adequate. We also enquired about part-time work for me, and although there was none available at that time it was probable that there would be by the time we moved north.

We saw an architect and gave him our ideas about the house we wanted to build on the ruins of four derelict crofts half way down the cliff overlooking one of the most beautiful harbours in the north of Scotland. After the building of the house started in 1969, I had a major operation and following this had another period of weakness of both legs and my right arm. At that time I was working full time and I managed to keep going for a year doing my own work, extra work for somebody on study leave and looking after the children and house. I became increasingly fatigued and in the end had to ask for time off work. At that time I was so exhausted and low that I was sent to a psychiatrist. I did not have any physical examination but was admitted to a nursing home for psychiatric treatment. I remember that I spent the first week asleep in bed and said that it was very like a physical illness. I was reassured that depression has that effect.

We had our usual holiday in the north of Scotland in 1970 and I was then recovering from my fatigue. I can remember now but did not draw attention to it at the time that I had great difficulty walking on uneven ground and down cliff paths. I was embarrassed because I fell over frequently for no apparent reason.

We fixed the date of our move north in August 1973 which seemed the least disturbing time for the children to move schools. I knew at the time that I should be in the north for a year before my husband retired. What I did not know was, that six months after our move north, he would take over as Chairman of his firm and that he would still be living in the south and I in the north more than five years later. It is as well that I did not know in 1973 that I should be a single parent with three teenage children for quite so many years and with so many other problems ahead.

My relatives and friends all thought that I was completely mad to be party, let alone instigator, to this upheaval. However, they were sure that I should not stick it out and would be south again within a year. They will never know just how often I agreed with their forebodings during that first, long, dark winter in the north. I had to help the children settle down at school, cope with an unfinished house, keep up my own morale which I found more difficult without a job and without my many friends in the south and try to adapt to a very different way of life. Indeed there were days when had some kind benefactor offered me a free move south I should have accepted it with alacrity. I just plodded through one day at a time and when I felt particularly low reminded myself that it had been almost impossible to get our small grand piano down the path when we moved into the house and it would be quite impossible to get it up again! However, we survived and in May 1974 I started working half time again which helped me a great deal.

In October of 1975 I went to East Africa for two months for a working trip with my husband. I had all the necessary inoculations before we went. It was a very busy trip and with a great deal of travelling. We spent much of the time on sisal plantations and sometimes walked down river banks to look at the disposal of the sisal waste. It is an area of Africa heavily affected by malaria and I was bitten by mosquitoes on many occasions. I did not worry because we were taking the recommended antimalarial tablets before, during and after the trip and never missed a dose. After our return and a fortnight after taking the last antimalarial tablet I had a sudden and very unexpected attack of fever. I had a second and more severe attack about ten days later and on that occasion I did see our doctor who took a blood smear and sent it to the laboratory. Nothing was found, which was not surprising, because the laboratory is 120 miles away! Between the attacks I forgot about the problem. After the New Year of 1976 I had severe attacks on two nights in succession. I thought that I must have malaria but it seemed an unlikely diagnosis in Caithness in mid-winter and I was sent to hospital in Inverness for investigation.

When I was examined in hospital there were some odd findings in my nervous system but presumably because they had no bearing on a mysterious fever after a stay in the tropics, nothing was done about them. I was very relieved because I had wondered if I should have a lumbar puncture. The diagnosis of malaria was confirmed and I went home again with lots of tablets to take. I should have been feeling better because all I was supposed to have was malaria and that was now under control. I felt so far from well that I began to think I must be mentally ill. I began to remember things that had been wrong for quite a while but seemed so trivial that I was sure I was making them up. I became so exhausted and depressed that once again I nearly went to a psychiatrist. However, in a moment of determination I asked if I could see the local consultant physician. He was kindness itself and listened to my string of apparently unrelated problems patiently. I felt a fraud and a hypochondriac to be bothering anybody with all these trivial matters. His examination confirmed that my complaints of things wrong were not all in the mind. There were too many physical signs of which I had known nothing.

The consultant found various things wrong with my left arm and thought at first that I had a localised neuritis. I had X-rays and tests but within a week my left foot started dragging. I did have some signs in the nerves of the right side of my head but because the main problems seemed to be on the left side of my body further tests had to be done to rule out anything unpleasant in my brain. I had an electroencephalogram, brain scan and other sophisticated tests.

When the 'non-invasive' investigations had been finished I

was admitted to hospital for one night for the 'invasive' investigation—a lumbar puncture. By this time both my legs were feeling very heavy and dragging when I walked. The signs in my nervous system had become more marked and before I left hospital the physician saw me and told me it must now be assumed that I definitely had multiple sclerosis. Of course, I heard him and I suppose I could say that I understood him, but it meant absolutely nothing to me. I think I had a feeling of relief that I should not now be sent to a neuro-surgical unit far away for even more investigations, the thought of which had horrified me.

I had taken two days off work for the lumbar puncture and then I started work again and tried to pretend that nothing had happened. I do not think that I had any intention of receiving any possible treatment or of taking any time off work. I went home to the children and said nothing about the illness. I did not telephone my husband about the diagnosis and, in fact, I did not tell anybody at all. I spent two nights awake trying to take it in but I think I intended to carry on as though nothing had happened. I do not remember feeling particularly anxious but stunned and in a slightly trance-like state. I can also remember vividly the ache up the back of my head and neck after the lumbar puncture. A car crash brought me to my senses. Luckily it was my car that was badly damaged and I was the only person hurt. Having driven for twenty-eight years without as much as a parking ticket, the incredible psychological jolt was enough to make me face facts.

I was taken by the police to the physician at the hospital, who took me and the children home and arranged for our general practitioner to come in and see me. I was mildly concussed and the headache kept my mind off other problems. Our general practitioner, while he was at the house, told the children what was wrong with me in a formal way and said that I should be staying at home for a while and might need some help from them. I realise now that the car smash was a merciful end to my folly and jolted me into accepting what help was available.

I spent nearly two months at home, mostly on my own, and had time and peace to recover from the shock of the diagnosis and acclimatise myself to the changes which were bound to take place in my life. I knew there was no real treatment for multiple sclerosis but was grateful for the palliatives I was offered. For three weeks I was unable to write and this I found very disturbing; luckily it passed.

During the following months I could gradually piece together the incidents which led up to the diagnosis and then realised that I had probably had the disease for many years in a fairly benign form with long remissions. In March 1975 I had been working in the local children's hospital and had caught some sort of virus infection which lasted about a month. After I got better I had aching shoulders and also found that my left hand was very clumsy and was inclined to shake. I had found this very embarrassing, especially first thing on Monday morning, when one of my jobs was to give the gynaecological consultant some help in the theatre. As soon as I had to hold a retractor with my left hand it started shaking. I thought the consultant would think I had taken to the bottle and found ways to rest my wrist so that the shake was minimised. After any strenuous effort with my left hand it was quite impossible to do any fine movements with it for some hours. It did cross my mind on one occasion that the clumsy shaking left hand could be due to multiple sclerosis but I forgot about it almost immediately and never let the thought back into my mind. The aching shoulders, the heavy feeling in my arms and my clumsy left hand went on all that year. I realise now that during that time I dropped a great number of things which was unusual for me.

Twice during 1975 I was in a warm climate. In June I had a holiday in the south of France and hoped that my aching shoulders would get better. They got worse and I found it difficult to swim. I found that I felt exhausted if I stayed in the sun, and this was quite new for me. In October and November while we were in tropical Africa I again found that my shoulders and arms were more troublesome and my fatigue was out of proportion to the amount of travelling we were doing.

Gradually, more and more incidents have dropped into place. Having had the disease for so many years I should have

CHAPTER TWO

Multiple Sclerosis
as a Disease

I expect if you are told you have multiple sclerosis you will be as ignorant about the disease as I was. After the diagnosis was made many friends said it must be worse for me being a doctor because I knew so much about it. Perhaps I was lucky because my knowledge of neurology and neuro-anatomy had always been a little sketchy and just adequate for passing examinations and recognising abnormal signs in a patient. I had no desire to go to a textbook and look up the disease and, therefore, my knowledge about it has remained a little fragmentary. I think experts would agree that multiple sclerosis remains an enigma in many respects and that knowledge about the disease is constantly changing. I will try and put together some of the facts and theories about the disease but shall not attempt a 'textbook' description.

First, it is important to realise that multiple sclerosis is a widely differing disease in different people. A diagnosis of multiple sclerosis thirty or even twenty years ago was considered to be a pretty gloomy one. Over the past twenty or so years it has gradually been realised that there is apparently a milder variety which has been called benign multiple sclerosis. Occasionally, a patient has shown the early symptoms of multiple sclerosis and then no further symptoms at any time. *Symptoms* are those things of which a person complains such as tingling in an arm or weakness in a leg and *signs* are those things that a doctor finds on examination. A symptom may be so mild that a person does not see her doctor and, therefore, it is not known later whether there were any signs of disease at that time or not. One or two of those people who complained of

15

mild symptoms suggestive of multiple sclerosis and who did not develop any further symptoms, eventually died of a disease which was completely unrelated to multiple sclerosis. When the brain and spinal cord were examined after death the characteristic appearances of multiple sclerosis were found. This suggests that it is possible for an indefinitely long remission to occur in multiple sclerosis and during life it may appear that the disease is cured. For this reason alone it is probably a mistake to make a definite diagnosis of multiple sclerosis when the first symptom or symptoms appear whether there are signs or not. If the disease is going to take a very long benign course, a diagnosis of multiple sclerosis at too early a stage can cause unnecessary anxiety and apprehension about the future.

The number of people in a community having multiple sclerosis varies with the geographical position of that community. Near the equator the incidence is very low and it increases as one moves further from the equator. It is particularly common in northern and temperate climates. It may vary from one part of a country to another. This happens in Norway where it is lower in coastal areas and higher in inland areas. It also happens in the United Kingdom where the disease is most common in Caithness and the Orkneys. For some extraordinary reason the Faroe Islands were remarkably free of the disease until recently. The reasons for this geographical distribution have been deliberated by many learned medical and other people. It could depend on diet and this is discussed in more detail in Chapter Eight. It has also been suggested that it could be connected with general hygiene and there is the possibility of an early spread of a virus infection among the community that could act as some sort of immunity. It is interesting that you retain the likelihood of developing multiple sclerosis connected with the area where you lived before the age of sixteen years. If you move from a high risk to a low risk area before the age of sixteen years you will then have the chances of living in a low risk area but if you move after the age of sixteen you will then keep the chances of a high risk area.

European Mediterranean communities, who not only live in a warmer climate but who are predominantly Roman Catholics, are oil eating and wine drinking, have less chance of getting multiple sclerosis than their more northern neighbours who are more likely to be Protestant, fat eating and beer or wine drinking. Oil is a fat which is fluid at room temperature and fat itself is solid and it has been suggested that not only the dietary habit of eating oil rather than fat but also religion may play a part in the development of the disease. The more passive Roman Catholics of southern Europe may be less tense, driving, compulsive characters than their northern neighbours who tend to be more hard-working and self-driving people.

The virus theory for the cause of multiple sclerosis is attractive in some ways and the type of disease caused in the nervous system could fit in with a viral cause. Multiple sclerosis is not like some other infections where there is a clear-cut illness and sometimes immunity for life following the illness. On the other hand there are virus infections of humans such as herpes simplex which causes a cold sore. Most children have been infected by the virus before the age of five years. Many of them will apparently recover completely but others will have recurrent sores throughout life, often when they are tired, emotionally upset or exposed to sunlight. Apparently the virus remains quietly tucked away in the body and only shows its presence when other conditions such as fatigue upset the resistance of the person. Chicken-pox is possibly similar because after apparent recovery the virus may remain dormant for many years in some of the nerves near the spinal cord. Years after the attack of chicken-pox, often in association with another illness or emotional upset, the same person may develop herpes zoster or shingles. It has been suggested that a similar viral infection acting in the same way could be part of the cause of multiple sclerosis. There are a great number of possible viruses that could be involved including the measles virus. Research work is going on and if a virus is involved one hopes that it will not be too many years before it is tracked down. It may then be possible to prevent the disease developing in those at risk.

The body has ways of defending itself against invaders such as germs. This defence is useful because you produce an immunity against certain diseases, either because you have had the disease (this is natural immunity) or because you have been immunised (this is artificial immunity). Normally the antigens or defending cells that attack foreign invaders do not attack the other cells in your body because they have some way of recognising them as 'self'. Sometimes, however, this method of recognition breaks down, the body fails to recognise 'self' cells and attacks them as enemy ones. This is known to occur in one sort of thyroid disease called Hashimoto's thyroiditis and it is thought that it may occur in other diseases such as diabetes and some sorts of arthritis. Now it is believed to be a possibility in multiple sclerosis; almost certainly not the whole story but possibly a part of it.

There is a possibility of a genetic or inherited factor in the development of multiple sclerosis. Close relations of someone with multiple sclerosis are estimated to be fifteen times more likely to develop the disease than those who are unrelated. There are also certain blood characteristics in the relatives of somebody with multiple sclerosis. This does not mean that multiple sclerosis is infectious and can be spread around the family. Neither does it mean that those in the family who are healthy should not have children. It is very easy to pick up a fact and distort it to the point where a life or lives are changed. There are so many unknowns in the cause of multiple sclerosis and any way of inheriting it is as yet so uncertain that there is no reason for close relatives to refrain from having children. For the young married woman who has multiple sclerosis the problem is rather different because it is her health that must be considered. Again there is no clear-cut pattern of pregnancy and childbirth making the progress of multiple sclerosis worse or better. Obviously one would not choose to become pregnant during a period of relapse but deciding never to have children may not be in the best interests of the husband or the wife. Looking back I can see that I had two episodes of multiple sclerosis during child-bearing but fortunately the progress of the disease has been slow and my life would have been much less rich without the family.

The individual patches of disease in multiple sclerosis are in the brain and spinal cord. They are not in the nerves of the arms or legs where the symptoms may occur. Each nerve has a central bundle of nerve fibres and is surrounded by a sheath which is called the myelin sheath. This sheath is made up mostly of fatty material part of which is fat called polyunsaturated fat. In multiple sclerosis the myelin sheath is damaged and under the microscope the reaction looks like inflammation. The damage usually starts near a very small vein and it has been suggested that whatever causes the damage may be brought in the blood stream. This would fit in with both a viral disease and what is called an auto-immune reaction where cells do not recognise 'self' cells.

At the time of the breakdown of the nerve sheath there is some swelling in the nerve and in the surrounding parts. There is also an increased number of white blood corpuscles in the area. After this initial reaction, during which there will be a variable amount of interference with the action of the nerve affected, the destructive process stops and the swelling goes. It is said that the nerve sheath cannot be repaired but always scars; now it is believed that a limited amount of repair may be possible. The signs of damage to the nerve itself often become completely absent although they may reappear permanently or temporarily at a later date.

These lesions seem to appear on the brain and the spinal cord in places where they are in contact with the cerebrospinal fluid (C.S.F.). This fluid circulates through the ventricles, small spaces within the brain, and around the brain and spinal cord. During life it may be possible for a doctor to guess at what position the lesion is situated by the signs it produces but often if the brain is examined after death, the damage may be more extensive than the signs would have led the doctor to expect.

The swelling caused by the reaction in multiple sclerosis may be particularly important at places where nerves pass through narrow bony canals in the skull. More damage may be done to the nerve if the swelling continues for any length of time than it would if there were space around the damaged area. The use of steroids in the early and acute stages of the disease or in an acute relapse probably reduces this swelling, and it has been suggested that this is their main use.

The start of multiple sclerosis may be so insignificant that at the time a doctor may not be seen and the diagnosis may only be made in retrospect after a further incident or incidents. Multiple sclerosis can, on the other hand, start more dramatically and the person be unmistakeably ill. The eventual outcome does not always depend on the acuteness of the onset. The illness is more common in women than in men and may start at any age from the teens onwards. The so-called 'late onset' which seems to start in the forties and fifties is possibly not a different type of illness but the manifestation of a relatively benign type of multiple sclerosis in which there have already been a number of minor episodes. At the time these may have been misdiagnosed or possibly no diagnosis has been made because the person never saw a doctor. It is quite impossible to give a description of typical multiple sclerosis because the disease is characterised by its infinite variability.

The first symptom may be in the eyes, with blurring of vision in one or both eyes and possibly some pain. This is due to a lesion in the optic nerve and if a patient is examined at this time with a light shone into the eye by an ophthalmoscope, a whitening may be seen of the optic disc at the back of the eye. This disc is the end of the optic nerve. If the lesion is in the optic nerve just behind the disc it may be possible to see that the disc is swollen. At this time vision may not only be blurred but there may be an absent patch of vision in the middle of the normal range of sight. Diplopia or double vision may be the first symptom of multiple sclerosis. Neither of these eye problems, although suggestive of multiple sclerosis, makes the diagnosis a certainty and it seems to me quite reasonable, even if the diagnosis should be suspected at this stage, that it should not always be disclosed. There may well be a period of many years before other symptoms appear and in the absence of any proven cure or method of preventing a relapse, a doctor could be well advised to keep his suspicions to himself.

Another early symptom may be either weakness or altered sensation in one or more limbs, most commonly a leg. The weakness may be felt as a heaviness and difficulty in lifting a foot off the floor or using a hand. The use of a hand may be so upset that it is called a 'clumsy' hand. The changes in sensation can be tingling or a feeling of a tight band, numbness or feelings of cold. If the limbs are examined at this stage there may be little to find and the amount of weakness which can be demonstrated is often less than the patient feels. This is a characteristic of the disease and not a proof that the patient 'is putting it on'. The tendon jerks in the affected limb or limbs may be slightly increased and there may be slight loss of a sense of touch and also of vibration as shown by putting a tuning fork on a bony part of the end of a limb. Sometimes, in apparently more severe forms of multiple sclerosis, there is an early loss of balance and there may be severe giddiness and vomiting.

Very often the first symptoms disappear completely although there may still be slight signs of disease on examination. Sometimes it is as many as twenty years before there are further symptoms; on the other hand, there may be more symptoms after only a few months. It is said that the longer the interval between the first and the subsequent symptoms, the better the outlook. This is very difficult to estimate because the original symptoms may have been present many years previously and been overlooked.

At some point in the course of the illness there are frequently bladder symptoms. These can be relatively mild and take the form of finding it necessary to pass water as soon as one has the urge. The bladder symptoms can be more severe and eventually result in failure to control the passage of urine.

If and when symptoms do reappear they may be the original ones that come back or, more commonly, others are added. They can include unsteadiness in walking, a tremor or shake in either or both hands, changes in sensation in the body as well as the limbs, and often muscle spasm and twitching in an affected leg. Pain is not usually a marked feature but muscle spasms can be very uncomfortable. At times there may be difficulties with speech.

Multiple sclerosis euphoria is described as the failure of a person to realise the nature of the illness. I have neither experienced euphoria nor met any other person with multiple sclerosis who has. Depression is much more common and often out of proportion to the severity of the illness at the time. Fatigue is a very common complaint and there is also a general loss of stamina in both physical and mental spheres. Depression may be increased by fatigue and relieved by physical and mental rest.

The diagnosis of multiple sclerosis is very often problematic because, although many tests have been devised, none is completely specific for multiple sclerosis and able to give a definitive answer. The history of symptoms getting better and worse over months or years or even varying in the course of a day may be suggestive. The examination of a patient who shows definite, although possibly slight, physical signs which could only be caused by more than one lesion in the central nervous system may also be suggestive. The cerebrospinal fluid may be examined after a lumbar puncture is done. This test means a minimum stay of twenty-four hours in hospital and is done with a local anaesthetic. It can show various changes including alterations in the cells present and the type of protein; there are other tests but none is a final proof of multiple sclerosis. More recently evolved tests measure the time of a response to light through the optic nerve. This is called the visual evoked response (V.E.R.). A similar test can be done with the auditory nerve. All the examinations and tests add up to give a general picture of multiple sclerosis and this, to a trained observer, means that the diagnosis is probable. Other diseases must be ruled out, including pernicious anaemia with involvement of the nervous system. This is a treatable disease and can be diagnosed with certainty.

There is no proven cure for multiple sclerosis and at the moment anybody who claims to provide one is either a victim of his own credulity or a deliberate quack. This does not mean, however, that nothing can be done to relieve symptoms and help with problems. It does mean that you should not leap at a promised cure by a course of injections unless they are a recognised part of research in which case the whole matter should be explained to you.

Steroids in the form of adrenocorticotrophic hormone

(A.C.T.H.) injections do seem to help in acute stages of the disease, particularly when vision is first affected. There is no evidence that prolonged courses of steroids do any good and they will make you liable to suffer from some of the unpleasant side-effects of the drug. Medicines may help with bladder problems, giddiness and muscle spasms. Advice from a physiotherapist can be helpful in strengthening weak muscles, relieving muscle spasms and preventing immobility in a limb. Rest seems to be important both in an acute episode and also in the long-term management of the illness. Complete bed rest is sometimes advised in an acute episode but personally I am nervous of spending more than an hour at a time lying down before taking a little exercise.

At the time of writing, the non-animal fat diet is widely recommended with additions of linoleic acid taken as sunflower seed oil. There are still some people following the much publicised gluten free diet but there is no medical evidence that it helps. When one studies the so-called gluten free diet as advocated by its devotees one finds that possibly animal fat, purified sugar, alcohol and coffee are also restricted. This rather detracts from the argument that gluten is the harmful substance.

It seems to me that much of the currently approved medical management has a common theme and that is physical fitness. Restriction of animal fats is being advocated in other degenerative diseases and exercise without exhaustion can do nothing but good. There is evidence that emotional upsets may be harmful in multiple sclerosis and avoiding them as well as mental and physical fatigue can be a lot more difficult than sticking to a diet. Whatever the management recommended, medical optimism, within the bounds of reality, is very helpful.

There are other less widely used and in most cases experimental lines of treatment. These include ways of suppressing the body's immune reaction which would be advisable if multiple sclerosis were an auto-immune disease. There is also a stimulator which can be implanted near the spinal cord and which seems to improve the symptoms in the legs and bladder. At the moment this is very costly, and its use severely restricted.

CHAPTER THREE

Some Medical
and Patient Mythology

Everybody knows that many patients hold myths about doctors and illnesses, and I think it is true to say that many doctors hold myths about patients and probably about illnesses too. Myths are more common with an illness that is both difficult to diagnose and has no established treatment; multiple sclerosis is included in both of these categories. Multiple sclerosis by its very nature, the doubts and difficulties in diagnosis, and the problems of its management, attracts a great deal of mythology and this neither helps the person with multiple sclerosis to accept and live with his illness, nor the doctor in helping his patient in as realistic a way as possible.

Most doctors are in the medical profession because they want to deal with illness and cure it if possible. Many doctors find it hard to accept that an illness is beyond their control and cannot be eliminated. Incurable illness and death possibly seem almost like a rejection to many doctors because they are left powerless. Perhaps doctors overestimate the effectiveness of medicines, operations and other forms of treatment, and underestimate the good that they can do just by personal contact with the patient as another person. I think many doctors have grown up with a feeling that it is dangerous to become over-involved with any patient and his problems. They feel that provided they can deal with the problems by medicines, that is fine, but if this is impossible they tend to feel that there is no value in offering friendly encouragement and understanding, and that it would be unwise to do so.

Possibly this is why one still hears from reliable sources of somebody having multiple sclerosis diagnosed and being told by a specialist that there is no point in his returning for another visit because there is nothing to be done about it. While I am sure this is rare, I have heard myself of instances when it has happened. It is, up to a point, true but sadly the doctor is under-estimating the power he still has of being able to counsel and help. Even if the follow-up appointment is at a year's distance it does mean that the patient will have the rare occasion to talk over his progress and his problems. It also means that should any further developments take place in the management or treatment of multiple sclerosis the doctor will not have lost contact with the patient. I think that a doctor who dismisses a patient with multiple sclerosis as incurable is possibly losing the opportunity of using a currently approved regime of management which will almost certainly help a person's morale even if it does not affect the outcome of the multiple sclerosis. I once worked for a doctor who said that 'pontification' was an occupational hazard of the medical profession. (Pontificate is to 'assume the airs of a bishop, to act dogmatically or pompously'). I certainly am not suggesting that doctors should be encouraged to act in this way. They should not, however, forget the authority they can use gently when advising a certain regime or giving advice on a life style, as well as the cautious optimism which they can show and which can be very encouraging.

There are doctors who have what may be described as a fanatical belief in one particular diet or regime. Not only may they become blind to other ideas and other developments but they can, by so doing, put too much onus on to their patients. For a time, if the patient is improving, all is fine; the doctor believes more firmly in his theories and the patient feels success at achieving the goals which are set. If the patient has a relapse there may be the inference that she is responsible, because she has in some way slipped from the regime or has not been playing her part with sufficient zeal in carrying out her doctor's instructions. Possibly such patients do not continue to attend the same doctor and such a doctor may be very much more aware of the 'successes' he is having than the 'failures'. In these cases a doctor of this sort may overestimate the effects of the regime he is prescribing, and underestimate the power that his determined personality has in keeping a patient well and active. The conclusions which he draws about the success of the regime he is advocating may not be very balanced; the publicity he may get, not only from his writings but from his satisfied patients may ultimately hamper rather than encourage a more rational approach to the management of multiple sclerosis. I am *not* trying to discourage anybody from following a recommended regime. Any regime which includes rest, diet and exercise is likely to help a multiple sclerosis patient to lead a more ordered life and to become generally fitter; this can do nothing but good. Fanatical belief in a regime may, however, lead to disillusionment and great discouragement if an improvement does not occur or if there is a relapse.

Many medical experts on multiple sclerosis would probably agree that multiple sclerosis is most likely to be wrongly diagnosed as a psychiatric illness or psychoneurosis. This does not mean that a doctor who fails to diagnose multiple sclerosis is negligent or in any other way at fault. It is often very difficult to make a correct diagnosis, particularly in the earliest stages of the disease. Even an expert neurologist may find little or nothing wrong. Nevertheless the disease may have started and once a patient has been labelled as neurotic it may be difficult for anybody to arrive at the correct diagnosis, even after repeated episodes and at a time when there would probably be some signs of disease if the nervous system were to be examined.

A non-medical friend made the statement that the medical profession seemed to act in the belief that a patient 'once a nutter is always a nutter'! While this is certainly not completely true and the word 'nutter' would not be acceptable to most doctors, there is a germ of truth in this comment. Once anybody, especially a woman, is diagnosed as having a psychiatric problem, it will take a very alert and all-seeing doctor to suspect that underlying the mental problems there is a physical illness. When further symptoms occur in multiple sclerosis it is all too easy to attribute them to anxiety or depression and treat them or dismiss them accordingly. The sufferer may have had a physical examination at the time of her very first complaints of illness but it is quite possible that there will not be further physical examinations if the same symptoms come back or if others occur. Should the symptoms suggest a psychiatric illness severe enough for hospital admission, the patient will then probably have a thorough physical examination and one hopes that the physical illness would come to light. On the other hand if a psychiatrist is seen as an outpatient or even privately there may not be any physical examination. It could be many years before the true cause of the problem comes to light. During this time not only does the patient fail to benefit from a more ordered way of life but he or she may suffer the problems both in her family, among friends and at work which can arise from a diagnosis of mental illness, even in these more enlightened days. Great harm can be done to marital relations in such a situation.

Possibly a misdiagnosis is likely to occur in multiple sclerosis not only because of the nature of the illness but also because of the personality of the patient. It is certainly a widely held belief, if not a confirmed fact, that multiple sclerosis sufferers have certain characteristics in common. Many of them are energetic and hard working, possibly to the point of overworking. Many of them tend to do things with bursts of energy. As the disease develops and fatigue begins to play a more prominent part this energy may become much less effective, and frustration and depression may result. Of course such depression can easily be mistaken for the cause of the illness rather than the result, and understandably so. I think that if you believe that you are tired and depressed *because* you are ill, and not ill because you are depressed, you must be prepared to take a firm stand with your medical adviser.

It is possible that the very fact of having had a psychiatric illness diagnosed tends to make anybody keep quiet about further symptoms which develop. If one can manage to keep going it seems better to keep them to oneself rather than be exposed to the seemingly inevitable label of being neurotic and a hypochondriac. This is a natural instinct and I know from personal experience that it happens. Others have told me that they do it, and I know there are occasions when I will still not admit, far less tell anybody, about a new symptom. It does not help your doctor and it probably does not help you.

Many doctors hold strong views about telling patients the nature of their illness. When the diagnosis of multiple sclerosis is first considered many doctors feel that the person should not be told. The first symptom may be of blurred vision of one eye or transient tingling in an arm or leg. There may be mild signs of disease at such a time but it is possible that the disease will progress no further. It is not finally known if there is a type of multiple sclerosis which is self-limiting. At the first incident it could be a mistake to tell the patient that she has multiple sclerosis because it might cause needless worry and suffering. On the other hand a patient may say at a later date, if the disease does progress or recur, that she should have been told earlier. This could be true for one person and untrue for another. If there was a proven cure for multiple sclerosis it might be very wrong not to be open about the possible diagnosis at an early date. Multiple sclerosis is not like that and if there is doubt about the diagnosis it could be better to let the patient remain unburdened by the thought of having multiple sclerosis.

At a time of recurrence of the symptoms and at a time when there may be more definite signs, the problem of telling or not telling the patient of the now likely diagnosis may become even more difficult. A doctor has to decide if his patient really wants to know that she has multiple sclerosis or if she would prefer to be told that she has something else wrong with her such as peripheral neuritis. What do the words 'multiple sclerosis' mean to her, and will she go to pieces if she is told the probable truth? The doctor may discuss the problem with the husband or wife or other close relative before making a decision. There are other people, and I am one of them, who would hate not to be told the truth, and are far more able to tackle problems once they are out in the open than try to cope with only the shadows of problems. If you feel that some part of the truth is being kept from you it will be partly up to you to make it clear that you do want to know the truth and will be able to accept and cope with it.

Some Medical and Patient Mythology

There are also myths held by patients about both doctors and multiple sclerosis. You may range from believing that doctors are all powerful and can do no wrong, to the opposite extreme that they are an arrogant lot and can be of little use! Doctors *are* human and the truth about most of them probably lies somewhere between the two extremes. When learning to accept and live with a long-term and variable illness like multiple sclerosis it is vital to have a doctor whom you trust and to whom you can turn in times of great difficulty. On the other hand you have also to learn to cope with your own problems to a large extent and be prepared to take your own decisions. It is tempting at times of uncertainty to lean too heavily on a doctor and then possibly blame him for things that go wrong. Doctors can give advice but not work miracles. It is up to you to take a responsible part in the management of your own illness, especially one with a prolonged course like multiple sclerosis.

I had my own private myth about neurologists which may be shared by others who are not medically trained. While I was a medical student I attended lectures and clinics given by a brilliant neurologist who was a consummate artist in the demonstration of abnormalities in the nervous system. I think my myth about neurologists arose at this time and I believed that they were brilliant academically but very much more interested in the physical signs of disease than in patients as people. I concluded that this attitude arose from their relative lack of power to control a disease of the nervous system in many instances. When a medical friend from 'down under' tried to persuade me to see a neurologist after the diagnosis of multiple sclerosis was made, it was several months before I could really bring myself to think about it seriously. Before I finally contacted the neurologist he had recommended I must confess that I got a 'character reference' on him. I was quite certain that his medical expertise would be superlative but I was much more anxious that he should be an understanding person. I need not have worried because not only has he given me excellent medical advice but also great understanding, wise counsel and encouragement in times of difficulty. My myth that a neurologist has nothing to offer but accurate diagnosis has been completely exploded by his practical suggestions and repeated encouragement to live a slightly less strenuous life.

When a diagnosis of multiple sclerosis is made, a person or the family may go in one of two directions about treatment. With a little knowledge about multiple sclerosis it may be easy to get into a despairing state which imagines that there is no cure and therefore there is nothing to be done about it but await inevitable disablement. This is probably more likely to happen without positive medical direction and encouragement. At the opposite extreme the person and the relatives may refuse to accept advice on the management of the disease on better established lines; they may believe that if they try hard enough, travel far enough, and possibly spend enough money, they are bound to find a 'cure'. Their search is going to be in vain and any temporary improvement from unorthodox methods could well be due to a spontaneous remission in the disease. Moving house just to be nearer a centre of research or treatment seems to me an unnecessary upheaval and more likely to do harm than good. Learning to live where one is and within the framework of an existing family and social pattern seems more important than to waste any effort chasing a promised but unproven cure. You can follow a sensible regime of living and try to keep physically and mentally fit whether you live near a medical centre for research into multiple sclerosis or many miles from one. I think it is more important that you make your existing life realistic than that you continually search for change which you believe could bring improvement.

When a remission does occur it is very easy to believe that the multiple sclerosis has got better and that you can now carry on living exactly as you did before you were ill. It is possible that you may be able to do just this for a few years or indeed for many years; if you are subjected to severe physical or mental strain it is quite possible that you will have a relapse. I think it is better to accept the fact that once multiple sclerosis has occurred, the scars remain in the nervous system and even if new damage does not occur when you get exhausted, old

CHAPTER FOUR

Acceptance

Acceptance of multiple sclerosis is very difficult to think or write about because it is not a finite act. Two years ago I could have said, and believed it to be true, that I had accepted the fact that I had multiple sclerosis, but I have discovered since that one continues to learn to accept different feelings and conditions as part of the same illness. Perhaps others are more clear-thinking and clear-feeling, and acceptance is for them a once and for ever process.

Although with hindsight it is now realised that I have had multiple sclerosis for many years, there was no question of acceptance until the diagnosis was made. When the diagnosis was finally made I was so shocked that it did not really mean anything. Probably in the first few days I hoped to remain an ostrich and carry on with my usual tactics of taking no notice and working rather harder. After the car crash, and when I finally stayed at home and rested, I remember feeling stunned with a very real sense of loss. The only time that I have felt this feeling before was when my father, of whom I was very fond, died.

It has been said by others that the diagnosis of any chronic and intractable disease such as multiple sclerosis can have the same effects as a bereavement. Bereavement has different effects in different people but seems to follow a fairly recognisable course. The first phase can be one of shock and bewilderment. There may be denial that anything has happened and a complete failure to realise its significance. I know that during the first weeks I felt quite numb and existed through each day in a mechanical sort of way. It was probably fortunate for me that all the children were at home and I continued going through the motions of getting breakfast, getting them off to school, pottering about the house doing a few chores and getting a meal for their return in the evening.

I had a great many letters, largely because my mother told many of our extended family and friends. I answered the letters, again in a trance-like state. I was commended for my courage—this I felt to be quite mistaken because I could not believe I was showing any courage while running away from the facts. I had become accustomed to using self-discipline through previous periods of ill-health. It was relatively easy for me both to lose weight and keep to a non-animal fat diet because of the long years when I had to discipline myself hard to keep going at all. The fact of keeping to a diet probably helped me during the early weeks because even in my stunned state I realised it was something positive to do. Possibly I developed an obsessive attachment to the diet and this helped to keep other problems out of my mind.

This initial stage of shock and stunned bewilderment is followed by a sense of realisation of the loss. This realisation may be accompanied by either the open expression of grief or with outbursts of anger about what has happened. Certainly I realised at some point that I had something wrong with me physically that would not go away and over which I had only limited control. I think the full implications and horror of becoming disabled only hit me and still does hit me when I am working and get so incredibly tired.

The idea of a body image is now widely accepted but was fairly new when I first heard a talk about it almost twenty years ago. I am not invariably impressed with new psychological concepts but this one impressed me at the time and I have remembered it. Two people who are both of more than average height can have entirely different views of themselves. I have seen this happen at very close quarters. My mother and I are exactly the same height but she would describe herself as a tall woman and I have never thought of myself as anything other than average height except when buying cheap dresses in chain stores! My own feelings about height seem to have been accepted by both my daughters who are fractionally taller than

I am but seem entirely happy with the image their bodies have for them. In the very early months of pregnancy, although there is no actual change in body size, the body image can change very much so that the pregnant woman feels quite a different shape. The reality and the image can be widely different.

I experienced this change in body image. Apart from clumsy hand movements and some difficulty in walking, especially in the dark or on uneven ground, nobody would have noticed anything wrong with me; yet at that time *I* had sudden and repeated views of myself as maimed and disfigured. There were times when I felt a very real revulsion for myself and felt that everybody must feel as revolted by me as I was. These very negative feelings caused depression and sometimes an almost paranoid feeling that I must be disliked by everybody because of the physical change in me. It is easy to dismiss this as the foible of an unbalanced mind but I have discussed this problem since with a woman in a very similar position, and again with no visible disability, and her experiences and mine are almost identical. Looking back one can see the lack of reality in this conception of oneself but at the time it was very real indeed. This period of depression over the change in my body image passed, but at times it has returned and for a while caused as much suffering as it did originally. Gradually I reconciled my mentally conceived body image with reality. The reality was that I was slimmer than I had been for twenty years and with no visible signs, at least to the casual observer, of disability. After I had the opportunity to re-equip myself with a considerably smaller size in clothes and found pleasure in borrowing my daughter's clothes, my negative feelings became less. I lost my sense of revulsion and regained my self-respect as a slim woman instead of as a considerably overweight one. I am aware that these are superficial feelings, and there is a real problem in this mental attitude towards disability which I will talk about again in Chapter Fifteen.

I did not consciously feel anger or bitterness about having multiple sclerosis, but probably these were feelings that I could not allow myself to experience. I might have felt better if I had.

I could have felt angry that the diagnosis had not been made many years previously when it might well have been, if I had been seen by a neurologist instead of a psychiatrist. There is no doubt that this misdiagnosis caused me a lot of difficulty and even suffering but on the other hand I could not have believed that an earlier diagnosis would have changed the course of the illness of multiple sclerosis a great deal.

In retrospect I think my anger was directed against myself thereby causing periods of depression instead of being directed outwards against some convenient medical figure. I can only guess, but I think my overdependence on doctors in the early months was also a queer way of showing my angry feelings. I know that anything I was told to do became a matter of law and I had to achieve any goal that was laid down for me including the one of weight. I became easily agitated and alarmed by trivial events and expected medical help to sort out problems which in my normal frame of mind I should have managed alone. Now it is reassuring to know that medical help is available should it be necessary. Perhaps in a sense I was taking it out on doctors—different doctors—who had in many ways in previous years 'taken it out' on me.

The third stage of a typical reaction to bereavement is said to be one of apathy; this I do not remember experiencing. By the time I was back at work and had recovered a little from my dejection and period of mental confusion, there were so many problems to be solved each day that I would have been unaware of apathy. The times since when I have come nearest to it have been those when I have felt intensely isolated and lonely, and lacked the energy to do anything about it. I live in an isolated place far from old friends and relatives and I was and often am alone, but when well I never feel either lonely or isolated. Now that travelling is becoming increasingly tiring I can see that contact with old friends will be more difficult and these patches may well increase. While there are always people with whom to make contact and things of interest to do here, these actions do need a certain amount of initiative and drive. At recurrent intervals I have neither. Strangely enough at the worst times I have often had a totally unexpected telephone call or letter which seems almost like an answer to an unexpressed cry for help.

The fourth and final stage of bereavement is described as readjustment, rehabilitation and acceptance. This stage I certainly went through and, indeed, continue to go through it, particularly after times when the going is tough. I found that I made a sort of mental balance sheet of what I had lost and what I still had to my credit. I had to do a great deal of mental spring cleaning and sort out those things in my life which were of real importance and jettison some undertakings and ambitions which were of less value. I am beginning to realise that many of my initial judgements were fanatically hard and that perhaps I should be better if I allowed myself a few more of the interests which give me pleasure without being too tiring.

In making my mental balance sheet I realised that I might well have lost longevity. This did not greatly bother me and I realised that I should be happy to be around for another ten years to see my family through to independence. The expense of the children's education had always been my contribution to the family budget and while the possibility remained that my husband might retire I did not want to unload that responsibility on to him.

I realised that loss of my mobility was a possibility but again this did not worry me unduly. I should be sorry to give up travelling but while I still had family ties I should not want, in any case, to run the risks of immunisations which can have a bad effect on multiple sclerosis. Otherwise the thought of my mobility did not worry me very much. I have been a bookworm since my early years and there has always been a collection of books waiting to be read. Less time spent rushing around and more time spent quietly reading could be a welcome change. I have many sedentary interests including a great fondness for listening to music and my large collection of records and good stereo could keep me happy for more hours in the day than I have to spare when mobile. In the past I have done a great deal of sketching and painting, and from the room where I should spend most of my waking hours, if less mobile, I have wonderful views over the sea, the cliffs and a fishing harbour.

While I was at home and my right hand was getting steadier I started playing around with pen and colour wash, and there is no doubt that the harbour views will provide many pictures!

My family must come first as long as they need me. I have realised that in putting my family first that there are enormous difficulties in keeping away from all thoughts of martyrdom. Adolescents do not want to feel grateful and neither do they want to know that a parent is existing primarily for them. Nothing must stop them from getting free and able to lead their own lives in their own way. In this direction I have made and continue to make many mistakes. I think it is important to learn a certain degree of selfishness so that they need feel no guilt in the pursuit of their own interests. I had to learn to say 'no' when asked to take on new commitments. Previously I had found difficulty in refusing a demand but now decisions could be made more clearly and at times more ruthlessly because there was a definite measuring stick. I have realised since that there is a very narrow margin between restriction of activity, which is good, and hibernation, which is bad and destructive of self and even of family.

I also had to do a physical spring clean because I found that life was simpler and less tiring if everything stayed in a reasonable place. Tidiness has never been one of my virtues and it is still very difficult for me to be orderly! However, it is worth the attempt because it is very much less tiring if one knows exactly where are the paper clips, kitchen knife, white cotton and the car keys. Effort spent looking for things is effort wasted and when fatigue is a constant problem, the expenditure of effort has to be spread very carefully.

I am sure that acceptance of an illness like multiple sclerosis is necessary before life can continue. Life can never go on as before but will have to progress more slowly and possibly in a different direction. It can take a long time to learn to achieve the things that are possible rather than habitually fail to achieve those that are impossible. The difference between the two will result either in growing happiness and a renewed sense of fulfilment or repeated frustration and despair.

You may say that acceptance is the wrong word to use and

the wrong attitude to take. 'One must learn to fight an illness such as multiple sclerosis'. I would agree with this if a fighting attitude is used in a constructive way towards rebuilding a future and surviving to the best of one's ability. I have seen a fighting spirit used in the wrong way antagonise doctors, family and friends and lead to many disrupted relationships and bitterness. Willpower and a fighting spirit can probably do little to control the disease in multiple sclerosis but if used rightly they can help in making the best use of mental and physical powers.

CHAPTER FIVE

Adjustments

Once you have had multiple sclerosis diagnosed and however well or minimally disabled you are at the time, there is little point in really believing that life can go on as before. Of course you want to be determined and optimistic and you are much more able to remain both of these things, as well as being a good wife and mother, if you can understand and be honest about the character of the illness that you have.

I think that most people with multiple sclerosis know what fatigue means. Most people without multiple sclerosis will also say that they are well aware of what fatigue means, but that is not quite the same. I can only try to explain that I and many other people with multiple sclerosis know that fatigue is different for us and for many of us it is the worst part of the illness. After I had been home for two months, in 1976, lost three stone in weight and managed to find a few clothes that about fitted me, I looked well, could walk fairly steadily and as I was right-handed, could cover up nearly all the clumsiness of my left hand. To all outward appearances I was well and healthy. At home I took regular daily exercise by walking up to the village and back, as well as going through my own personal routine of exercises. I pottered about the house quite a lot, although at that time I had somebody who did the housework for me. I was indulging in what I then looked on as the luxury of an afternoon rest. I definitely had the feeling that I was swinging the lead more than a little and was restless to get back to work. My car had not been patched up but I bought an old one to tide me over and then asked for release from medical custody, which was given me.

I started back to work and was quite appalled about how

tired I got. I only work half time; I found I could manage half Monday and half Tuesday, but by Wednesday I was, to put it in my son's words, 'knackered'. I really hardly knew how to drag myself around. My walking was less steady and I found that having started to sit down on a chair I just dropped into it, which was singularly inelegant and quite worrying. At the time I did not really tie these things up with multiple sclerosis but felt that it was just the shock of returning to work after so long a rest and with a little patience and a lot of willpower this ridiculous fatigue could and must pass.

I curtailed all other activities apart from my half-time medical work, which is not particularly strenuous apart from the lengthy drives involved. I did some journalism to which I was committed. I did not go out in the evenings—I could not have managed it because, having got the evening meal, I was ready for nowhere but bed. I was often too tired to eat in the evening. The children were very good about clearing up the meal.

As the weeks passed my fatigue did not improve. It was always the same pattern. I did practically nothing on Saturday and Sunday. I managed quite well on Monday and Tuesday, Wednesday was a bit of a nightmare and the rest of the week was disastrous. I got gradually more tired and more irritable. I remember one Wednesday evening, coming in from what was by my standards a very light day, but feeling so frighteningly tired, that I felt I could not get through another day of work. I seriously wondered if this was all in my mind or whether it really could happen in multiple sclerosis, and if so I had not read much about it. I telephoned the welfare officer at the Multiple Sclerosis Society in London and told her my tale of woe. She was marvellously understanding and said that it was very common indeed, for those with multiple sclerosis, to feel as tired as this. She told me that it was fatigue rather than disability that caused most multiple sclerosis patients to give up work. I could well understand why. From that time I realised it was something that had to be admitted, adjusted to, and lived with because clearly, life as it was then, was not worth living and by being so constantly tired not only in body but also in mind I was unable to be an even reasonably competent mother.

Now, eighteen months later, I get less tired but I am sure this is because I have become more used to doing less. Sometimes I feel well and I forget for a while, work harder, and then suddenly find myself so utterly exhausted that I get depressed at my stupidity. It is a sense of failure and inadequacy that I can manage so little. I, like many multiple sclerosis patients, find travelling particularly tiring. I find for the moment at least that I have had to cut down even short business trips abroad with my husband because the exhaustion they cause, what with journeys, late dinners and constant movement, are just not worth the effort. I am very sorry about this and hope that perhaps later I shall be able to manage again.

What then are you going to do about daily living and daily working? I think that it is a good idea early in the illness while you probably have little disability and may be able to expect long periods of remission to think about occupation. I do not, however, think that it is pessimistic, to think about a future when you may be less mobile. Rather is it realistic. Of course, you hope that this will not happen to you or that it may be so many years distant that it is not worth thinking about. The problem will be different if you are the man who is the breadwinner of the family, and I will talk more about this in Chapter Thirteen.

Any housewife will probably say that she need never think about occupation! The hours are always insufficient in the day for all she has to do. If you feel this way I do not want to discourage you but I would suggest that you think a little about a less active existence in the future. A daily rest in the middle of the day is a very good idea and a habit which will probably stand you in good stead for the rest of your life. Of course there will be days when you cannot manage it, when there are things like school sports and other important occasions. I think that it is more important, if you can manage it, to attend such functions and respond to the demands of your family than stick to the routine that you know may be better for your health. You can always go to bed early in the evening and rest a bit longer the next day. You will not be able to see wee Ian win the hundred metres or the high jump again. It is a question of keeping things in proportion.

What are you going to do while you rest? Perhaps you can sleep which may be a very good idea. If you do not sleep it may be a good idea to start reading again; you may once have been an avid reader but the habit can easily be lost during the child-rearing years. When you sit down at all you have not the energy to concentrate on reading a book; then you reach the stage of skimming through a daily paper and floating gently through a weekly and possibly a monthly woman's magazine. Occasionally you indulge in the luxury of *Vogue* or *Harpers* that a wealthy friend has left behind after a visit! It might be a very good idea to start reading the reviews of books and pick out one or two that you think would interest you and get them from the library, or you can ask the librarian for a book that he thinks you will enjoy. You may prefer to return to a newer work of a former favourite author. It may even be a good idea to join one of the well-run book clubs now available and have the pleasure of choosing a number of books each year that you can afford to buy and have time to read.

Having started to read again you may even find that you feel like studying. Perhaps you might do a postal course in journalism or learn another language with a linguaphone course. I know one enterprising woman of over sixty with multiple sclerosis who has started a degree course with the Open University. You may prefer more passive occupations such as listening to music. It may help you to enjoy television and radio if you look through the programmes in advance and plan your rest to coincide with a concert that you really want to listen to.

If your hands are still mobile you may want to develop other skills such as dressmaking, embroidery, macramé work, lamp-shade making or a host of other interesting crafts. Writing letters is a fascinating occupation if you make the time for it; if you have clumsy or shaky hands you may find it much easier and less frustrating to use a typewriter than write by hand.

Have a look at your home and your garden. Are you going to stay in this home indefinitely or are you going to move? It is certainly a good idea to have a labour-saving house even if you are still fully mobile. Have you got easy access to your front door and could you get a car there if necessary? At the moment our garage and drive are at a much higher level than the front door and there are three flights of steps on the front path. I have already found that in a strong wind I tend to blow over on the steps, so we are going to have a handrail put along them. I have asked an architect friend to survey the levels and give advice on the possibility of a drive down to the front door, if it should become necessary. I do not call any of these plans pessimistic but realistic, because I should prefer to remain in this house where I have such a beautiful view over the sea and harbour. It is problems like steps and access that you need to watch when you are choosing a new house or having one altered.

There will probably be many passing physical problems and some permanent ones. These problems may include phases of blurring of vision or double vision, weakness in arms or legs or other muscles and sometimes trouble with passing urine. You will find that a new problem may come on or an old one come back when you are very tired and it can clear up again in a matter of days. It is important that you do not adopt an early philosophy of 'learning to put up with it'. This attitude may be fine if you are really disabled when to be able to accept disability cheerfully seems commendable. In the earlier days when something might be done, do *not* put up with your problems. It is surprising how often if you ask for help it really can be found in a number of different ways. At one point I was unable to carry a fairly large tray with anything on it. The tray always tipped to one side and whatever was on it rolled off, broke, and I felt very frustrated. For a while I just gave up carrying a tray. When I told an occupational therapist about the problem she lent me a sheet of marvellous adherent white material which stopped anything falling off should the tray tilt. The problem passed; the white miracle sheet was returned to the occupational therapist; I had learned that it was always worth trying to solve a problem rather than blindly put up with it. Sometimes exercises can help and at the moment I am seeing a physiotherapist about difficulties in sitting up for long because of an aching back. Possibly strengthening my back muscles will overcome this problem.

It is no good discussing a problem of this sort with anybody who has a 'you poor poor thing' approach. You do not want sympathy but you do want a fresh mind to tackle your problems. It will not necessarily be a doctor or other professional person who can help you solve a problem but could quite possibly be a friend with an inventive mind. The same difficulty in sitting up has made typing very tiring for me and uncomfortable. I just 'put up with it' and lay down flat every half hour or so until the discomfort had gone off. Now a neurologist has suggested that I should have my typewriter on a sloped wooden rest with a board in front. At the moment I have tried it with an old tray propped up on a pile of books. It has helped enormously and I can type for much longer periods. When I can manage to get a joiner to make a more permanent edition I shall not have to put up with the present instability of the pile of books!

Although you may realise that there is no medicine or treatment that you can have to make multiple sclerosis go away, it is worth asking your doctor for help with coping with a temporary thing like muscle twitching, cramps, giddiness, and sometimes problems with passing water. All of these problems may be helped temporarily and to some extent with tablets or medicines. In the long run nobody understands the progress of multiple sclerosis but in the short term there may well be some relief available for a troublesome symptom. In multiple sclerosis so many problems are passing and nobody will ever know whether the medicine made the problem go away or it just got better by some natural process of healing.

One of the most difficult things for some people with multiple sclerosis is learning to accept help. It is so much better if you can learn not only to accept help that is offered thankfully but also to ask for the help you need. You will find that often those closest to you really do want to help but just do not know what is necessary. If you are tired in the evening they may be very willing to wash up and tidy the kitchen for you if you ask them. If you do not ask and get exhausted it is your own fault, and it will not help anybody to feel martyred about it.

It is also worth thinking about labour-saving methods and gadgets. Amongst gadgets I would rank in importance a fully automatic washing machine and if you can afford to run it a tumble dryer. An automatic washing-up machine can be a great help if there are several of you in the family. A deep-freeze can be a great help in reducing shopping, for shopping can be very exhausting. You can buy meat in bulk and therefore afford some more expensive cuts. Roasting a large joint of meat saves work if you have cold meat for a meal or two. For cooking the cheaper cuts I have found that the new automatic slow-cooking pots save a lot of supervision in the kitchen. It is also very helpful if you have a heavy day to prepare the meal the night before. Turn on the switch before you leave the house in the morning and come home in the evening to a welcome smell of a meal all ready. Gallon cartons of ice-cream and refrigerated sauces such as chocolate and butterscotch to go with them spare a lot of time and energy in meal preparation, particularly if the numbers of people present are unexpectedly large. If you have no disability which makes driving difficult it is still worth while considering the future in buying a new car. Automatic transmission may help you to drive a lot longer if you have any trouble with your left leg. It is worth considering a diesel car if you can stand the increased capital outlay. The main advantage to a multiple sclerosis sufferer is that you need change gear very little. It is possible to go from ten miles an hour to seventy miles an hour in top gear with some diesel cars. Only a trial run will help you to decide the advantages for yourself.

I realise that some readers of this book may feel they could never afford some of these labour-saving gadgets which I suggest. May I also suggest that you discuss their purchase with the Social Services and, if help is not forthcoming, that you contact the Multiple Sclerosis Society. I shall be discussing this further in Chapter Seventeen.

CHAPTER SIX

Early Treatment

As soon as the diagnosis of multiple sclerosis is made you may either do as I did and pretend that nothing has happened and that business will continue as usual, or you can be more constructive and accept what medical advice is offered you. If the disease is in an inactive state and if you have possibly had it for a number of years when this is diagnosed, you may well not be recommended to have any special palliative treatment. You will probably be advised about rest and exercise and probably some supervision will be kept over your progress. It will be a good idea if you are sent to a physiotherapist to learn about suitable exercises which need to be tailor-made for your particular problems of the moment. Courses of intensive physiotherapy are usually of little value because you will find if you are attending a physiotherapy department you will be doing too much at one time and too little the rest of the week. Once you know the suitable exercises you will be better doing them a little at a time on your own at home. The main problem is that this approach needs self-discipline; it is better to start to learn now what you are going to need in the way of self-discipline over the years.

If the multiple sclerosis is diagnosed in an acute and early phase a varying degree of rest is bound to be recommended. Years ago complete bed rest was advised and some doctors still recommend this. I, as I have said elsewhere, am quite frankly frightened of staying in bed completely. It is possible that I should be better at times if I did but I have a quite definite notion, possibly unreasonable, that getting up, pottering around and doing a few exercises at least once an hour is the best insurance I have against becoming less mobile. There is no authoritative medical backing for my particular prejudices about this and I must emphasise that my forthright views have been implanted from within; none of them from without.

If complete or almost complete rest is advised the question of where it may be best achieved will have to be decided. A mother with young children may find it impossible to make arrangements so that she can get sufficient rest at home. It may be possible for her to go to her parents or it may be necessary for her to go into hospital for a while. I do know that rest in hospital is advised for a number of conditions but both as a doctor and a patient I often wonder why. Perhaps even more as a patient I am very well aware that a hospital is one of the least restful places in which to spend any time. Even in a single room there seems to be some sort of noise going on for most of the twenty-four hours. Too many of the doors have that devilish invention of a glass pane above them and invariably a light in the passage outside which is left on night and day. I have found that even if the peripheral noise abates, the light never stops, and it is difficult to get undisturbed sleep. There seem to be never-ending processions of drug trolleys, people wiping things that already look clean, medical rounds, office sister rounds, chaplains calling, good ladies selling things off trolleys, not to mention the paper and the post. If by chance I dropped off for a nap during the day, I always seem to have been woken up because somebody wanted some blood! Complete hospital rest is to me a myth and I'm not meaning to be funny. Possibly the most peaceful establishments are those run by religious orders!

I was fortunate because my children were able to be more or less self-supporting. I had somebody coming in to do the housework each day, and it was quite possible to stay at home and have a reasonable amount of rest. I never actually spent a whole day in bed and there was never a day when I did not get up and dressed for most of the time, but that did not mean that I was not able to enjoy a great deal of mental and physical relaxation. For me it was very much better to be at home because there was some little thing to do that kept my mind occupied, and anyway I always feel more at peace and secure in my own home. I could wander around and water my infinite variety of house plants, enjoy the company of the various domestic animals, indulge myself in listening to my favourite records and programmes of music and above all let my mind rest on the incredible beauty to be seen from the room where I spend most of my working days. I had a foot extension for my favourite chair and from there I could see the harbour, cliffs and sea. There is seldom a time during the day or night when there is nothing happening at the harbour, and this means that although our house is isolated I always have something or somebody to watch, and on which to focus my interest. I find it very much more relaxing to be able to make myself a hot drink when I want it, eat, write, to stick to my diet, but have things the way I like them. For me, rest has a strong streak of self-indulgence but for all that, after a few days rest at home I think I am able to show enough self-discipline and benefit more than after a much longer rest in hospital with an enforced discipline.

It is usual to have steroids at the start of multiple sclerosis or during an acute episode particularly if your eyes are affected. Steroids are usually given in the form of A.C.T.H. Other forms of steroids depress the steroids produced naturally by the body and may in the long run do less good. A.C.T.H. does not have this unfortunate depressing effect on the body's natural production of steroids. Unfortunately, A.C.T.H. cannot be taken by mouth and has to be given by injections. Every neurologist or doctor who treats patients with multiple sclerosis has his own particular way of giving a course of A.C.T.H. injections. A depot or long-acting injection is usually given and is normally given in fairly large doses perhaps every second day for the first week then every third day and gradually tailing off over three weeks. Some courses last longer than this but there is no evidence that steroids given over very long periods are of any benefit at all in multiple sclerosis.

Some people find that A.C.T.H. gives them a feeling of well-being and tends to increase the appetite. Actually I found neither. I continued to feel exceptionally tired and my appetite, already poor, disappeared completely. This could have been due to the shock of the diagnosis or of my own brain-washing in my anxiety to reduce weight. It is usual to put on some weight while having a course of A.C.T.H. but I continued to lose at a very rapid rate. Extra potassium should be taken while A.C.T.H. is being given.

During the short course of A.C.T.H. there are unlikely to be many of the unpleasant side-effects which steroids can cause, including weight gain. Care should be taken if the patient is known to have a raised blood pressure. During the last week I was on steroids I noticed that my face looked fuller and was rather flushed which can happen with steroids. I was also rather anxious to notice that some of the downy hair on the lower part of my face had darkened and seemed coarser. I had a brief vision of developing a moustache and side-boards but forgot about that. The down on my face is entirely normal now, so it must have put itself right, because I never did anything about it in the cosmetic way. At the time it was a passing anxiety because I had other things on my mind.

It is difficult to say whether A.C.T.H. causes any great improvement. Certainly my legs became much steadier and my walking better. A tremor of my right hand developed while I was having the injections and did not clear up until after they were finished. At the time I felt a great sense of relief that something positive was being done by having injections and that they might help. In the last weeks before I had stopped working the weakness and uncertainness of both my arms and legs had become worse at rather an alarming rate. It is impossible to know if the A.C.T.H. was responsible for the improvement, or if the peace and rest of a period at home had as much to do with it as the drug.

I suppose if I should have a severe relapse and be advised to have A.C.T.H. again I should agree, but I think I really have more trust in physical and mental rest. A.C.T.H. in a short course is relatively harmless but perhaps I have a natural suspicion of things which play around to some extent with my own hormone balance. I should certainly accept A.C.T.H. for affected eyes because I think in that case it can cause dramatic improvement. Eye problems in multiple sclerosis where the optic nerve is involved are probably the most important reason for giving A.C.T.H.

Some doctors prescribe injections of B_{12} and these may be given twice a week and continued for some months. There is no particular evidence that they do any good in multiple sclerosis but they certainly do no harm and are known to have a beneficial effect on nervous tissue in other diseases. I have never had B_{12} because the doctors treating me have not believed in it, but at odd times when very tired, I have occasionally wondered if such injections might not be a little beneficial or just have some magic about them. On the whole it is my impression that nurses are more in favour of the beneficial effects of injections of B_{12} on general health than are doctors.

In order to acquire rest of body and mind and to lessen the initial effects of the shock of the diagnosis you may be given a mild sedative. Many people prefer to manage without sedatives but if you are very tense and agitated, a short course of a sedative may help you rest. It is believed that emotional upset has a detrimental effect on multiple sclerosis, so that it is reasonable in treatment to be given something to help produce a relaxed body and mind. Valium can be a useful sedative; it can also help relieve muscle spasms which can sometimes be annoying and uncomfortable in the limbs. I have found that the spasms have on occasions been particularly troublesome at night, and Valium does seem to help the muscles relax and then make sleep more possible.

From the beginning of your time at home, I think you will find it helpful and reassuring to work out a daily routine. You do not have to stick to this routine rigidly but having some sort of plan for your day may help you to feel more secure. Set your mealtimes and plan your diet. Whether you are hungry or not, prepare and get your food at approximately the time you have arranged for yourself. Try not to drink too many odd cups of coffee and tea because they will tend to make you more tense and may interfere with your sleep. Make sure you have your mid-day rest even as you begin to get more active.

I found it helpful to have certain times of the day planned for writing letters and reading. My *Radio Times* became interesting reading because I could plan the programmes to which I really wanted to listen or watch. If you are going to get back to work within a certain time you want to start increasing your exercise and the amount of your general activity slowly and steadily. You can feel very strong and brave while you are doing very little and leading a very protected life; suddenly becoming more active and having to keep to a more rigid timetable with more demanding days can come as a great and tiring shock. I do not think there is any way of cutting out the fatigue when you start work again but at least you can mitigate it by breaking yourself in to a tougher life slowly and gently.

CHAPTER SEVEN

Multiple Sclerosis
and Diet

There are a number of people who have strong convictions that one or other sort of diet can produce a miraculous cure in multiple sclerosis. These passionate ideas are fostered by some of the popular press and particularly health magazines, who publish accounts either written autobiographically or skilfully presented by an interviewer, describing remarkable cures from following one particular diet or regime.

Probably the most dramatic of all is the still publicised account of a writer who developed multiple sclerosis and was partially crippled. He disappeared from the writing world and was later tracked down by a curious journalist. This man had put himself on a gluten free diet and also eliminated coffee and alcohol from his diet. According to the man he had made a miraculous recovery and was able to move about freely again, and to lead a full and normal life. Neurologists examined him and found signs that he had had multiple sclerosis but was indeed very well and mobile.

Following the first publication of this story there were, quite naturally, nationwide enquiries at neurological departments about this wonder cure. The neurologists knew nothing about it but many patients went on the diet because at least it could do them no harm and in a progressive illness for which there is no known cure it is wrong to deny patients any hopeful avenue of help. One neurologist undertook a trial of the gluten free diet with forty-two patients. Five patients dropped out of the trial because they found the food unpalatable: of the remainder who stayed on it for the length of the trial there was no evidence that their symptoms improved or that they were less likely to relapse. Following this trial few neurologists would recommend a gluten free diet to new patients but there are still many people who are trying this diet and a new recipe book for them has recently been published.

The gluten free diet is used primarily for children or adults who have coeliac disease; for them such a diet is essential for the rest of their lives. Gluten is the harmful part of protein in wheat, rye and barley and a gluten free diet means that all food taken should be without these cereals. Bread, cakes, biscuits and puddings must be made with gluten free flour and a careful watch kept on the ingredients of all foods used, such as tinned foods, sauces, ketchups and gravies. With great skill the specially baked foods can be reasonably tasty but not as tasty as food made with normal cereals. The person with coeliac disease knows that taking gluten is incompatible with good or even reasonably good health, and this in itself is usually sufficient incentive to remain on the diet. The patient with multiple sclerosis has no such medical certainty to help him keep to the diet, but if he feels passionately that such a diet will improve him few doctors would disillusion him. At least most people on a gluten free diet tend to lose weight because the food is not very appealing!

Two other arguments have been put forward in favour of the gluten free diet but both have been discounted. One was the high flour and therefore gluten intake in the north of Scotland and the Orkney Islands where multiple sclerosis is common. This area has the highest reported incidence of multiple sclerosis in the world; I say 'reported' because where any illness is thought to be common, it is more likely to be sought out and diagnosed. The idea of the illness is already in a doctor's mind and probably he is less likely to miss a case than in a place where the disease is a rarity. There has also been an idea that there might be some change in the intestine in multiple sclerosis similar to that in coeliac disease. Further examination of this idea has shown it to be untrue.

I will digress here to explain double blind trials to those who are not familiar with them. They are the nearest that the medical profession can get to experiments on human beings. Two sets of people are chosen who are matched as nearly as possible. In the case of multiple sclerosis they would be matched for the state of the disease and whether it is in an active stage. They would also be matched for age, sex, whether married or not and for anything else that seemed relevant to the trial. They would then be allocated without their knowledge, or the knowledge of the doctors controlling the trial, to a treatment group and to a control group. To make the matter even more scientific, both groups are given identical appearing capsules, tablets, diet or whatever else the trial is investigating.

At the end of the trial everybody is examined again and their progress recorded and in the case of multiple sclerosis any recurrences and remissions during the period of the trial are also recorded. It is only then that the doctors know who had the 'real' treatment and who had the 'imitation' treatment or a placebo.

In some trials it is found that as many people will improve with a placebo as with the drug undergoing a trial. Sometimes this can show the power that interest and suggestion can play in the relief of symptoms but in multiple sclerosis it probably shows that a spontaneous remission has taken place unconnected with any so-called treatment.

For obvious reasons a gluten free or a non-animal fat diet which I shall describe cannot be subjected to assessment by double blind trial because those in the trial would know very well if they were being given gluten free bread or if animal fat had been banned from their food. Doctors are naturally suspicious of claims about improvement in possibly only one or a few cases when patients have tried a special diet. This is particularly true in an illness like multiple sclerosis which has normal fluctuations over the years where it is very difficult to make claims which satisfy the medical profession about any particular line of treatment. At the time of writing there is medical support for the non-animal fat diet. Most doctors would concede, however, that neither diet would do any harm if used properly, and would give their blessing to either diet if the patient felt that it was doing him good.

The low or non-animal fat diet was first tried by an American,

Dr. R. L. Swank, who commenced his trials in 1948 and first published his work in 1959. Many neurologists and other doctors would now give him credit for this early work on what is now the most favoured diet. However, then and later he is criticised for publishing the results and basing a theory on relatively few treated patients. There have been several editions of his book describing his method of treatment and giving a number of recipes. The book is easy to read, encouraging and very illuminating if you can get a copy of it.

His first work on low animal fat diet was done at McGill University in Montreal in 1948. He had observed that in areas where the total intake of fat in the diet is less than 24 grammes (g) a day the incidence of multiple sclerosis was low. In areas where multiple sclerosis had a higher incidence the daily fat intake could be as high as 150g a day. He distinguished fats into hard fats which are set at room temperature and soft fats or oils which are runny at room temperature. In his first trial the limits on daily intake were 15g for hard fat and 20g for oil. He considered it apparent that oils did no harm and raised the upper limit of daily intake of oil to 50g after 1952.

While studying dietary habits Dr. Swank came to the conclusion that multiple sclerosis as well as other degenerative diseases has probably only been in existence for about 200 years. He could find no mention of a disease like it in the Bible, as we can with other long-established diseases. He came to the conclusion also, that people living in advanced and especially western countries had eaten an increasing amount of animal and butter fats particularly over the past two decades.

More recent studies on fat intake and multiple sclerosis have reached the same sort of conclusion. With certain exceptions the incidence of multiple sclerosis is lowest nearer the equator and increases the further one travels from the equator. Diets in general have more oils and less fats near the equator and more fats and less oils further from the equator. There are some interesting differences in the local incidence of multiple sclerosis which also seem to be related to dietary causes. For instance in Norway the multiple sclerosis incidence is higher inland than in coastal areas and this again appears to reflect the intake of oils as opposed to fats.

Oils and fats can be described more scientifically as saturated fats and mono-unsaturated fats or polyunsaturated fats. The difference is in the formula which is complicated; in the poly-unsaturated fats there are two or more carbon atoms linked together by a double instead of a single bond and this makes them more active in the body. The saturated fats are the animal fats and other fats which are solid at room temperature such as the more conventional sorts of margarine. It is the poly-unsaturated fats that appear to be desirable in people with multiple sclerosis. A number of theories have been put forward to account for this phenomenon but in general it seems that a higher concentration of polyunsaturated fat in the blood protects the nerve from whatever it is that starts off demyelination in multiple sclerosis. There are almost certainly other factors than the proportion of various sorts of fats in the blood.

If you do decide to try a non-animal fat diet, and many doctors would encourage you to do this, it is important to realise that you are trying an experimental regime and not embarking on a proven cure. I think it does make a big difference if you realise this because then you will not give up the diet in a month if you are not incredibly much better. It is essentially a diet with which you will have to live many years—possibly for your whole life and there is going to be no evidence that you would have been better or worse without it. You may have to give up food of which you are very fond and you will have to be prepared to do it thoroughly rather than just playing around with the diet. It may complicate your own and other people's lives and if you are only doing it half-heartedly it would not really be fair for either yourself or the reputation of the diet. *This is no crash diet but one that has to be lived with*; it is important to make it as acceptable to your palate as possible, and also to make it fit in with family cooking and eating as much as possible. On any long term diet, whether it is a redu-cing diet or a non-animal fat diet, it is less harmful if you must cheat at all to have one good cheat a month rather than three small cheats every day. At least that way your body will be getting the benefit of the diet for most of the time.

If you and your doctor decide that you are going to try a non-animal fat diet it is helpful to see a dietician to discuss it with her in detail. In general you should avoid completely the following: whole milk, butter, cream, margarine, cheese (except low fat cottage cheese), chocolate, lard, and anything which contains any of these foods. An average helping of lean meat may be taken once a day and eggs, if taken at all, should be limited to two a week. The white of egg can be eaten with restriction. Low fat cottage cheese and plenty of white fish should be taken to keep up your protein intake. Food where possible should be grilled rather than fried. Oil, when used for cooking or making mayonnaise or French dressing, should be sunflower seed oil. This oil is more expensive than other oils and can usually be obtained from health food or wholefood shops. If bought by the gallon it is cheaper. I find that nobody in the family notices any difference in taste and although it is more expensive I use it for all cooking including roasting, bread making, and French dressing. You can use margarine which is labelled as containing polyunsaturated fat either on your bread or in your cooking.

I found it easiest to go on to the diet straight away as soon as I had had it explained to me. For me, cheese was the hardest thing to give up and I have never dared cheat with it because I fear that like an alcoholic with alcohol, one small piece might start me off again, on an addiction of many years standing. I find that low fat natural yoghurt is a great standby for puddings and at other times. I have never found a satisfactory way of making my own yoghurt with skimmed milk and I therefore have a weekly order for fifteen tubs of yoghurt with a local grocer. It is far more expensive than making my own but far more delicious and I do indulge myself in this way!

Fats provide twice as many calories per gramme as either protein or carbohydrate; therefore, by cutting out the majority of fat from your diet you can, if you are not needing to reduce your daily calorie intake, find yourself taking an unacceptably low level of calories and you may become weak and tired as a result. To counteract this tendency you will probably have to increase the amount of protein and to some extent the amount of carbohydrate in your food. I found in practice that it is useful to use whole cereals and I started baking my own bread and making my own muesli which has proved more than acceptable to the entire family. Beans and peas, soya beans, textured vegetable protein and the newly developed sprouting seeds are all ways of increasing my daily protein intake. Sprouting seeds is an amusing and easy exercise and one that can be done in the kitchen or a sitting-room either with kilner jars or with one of the special American spherical devices. I have one of the latter and I am always amused by watching a visitor eyeing this for a while before asking me what my green and purple sphere is for. I find the sprouting seeds are delicious eaten raw as salad and the whole family enjoys them cooked with onions and tossed in soya sauce. In such ways one can make a diet for a lifetime into a very interesting pastime.

If you cut animal fat out of your diet and like me you do not enjoy any sort of margarine, you are going to be taking a diet deficient in vitamins A, D, and E. You will therefore need to take one multivitamin tablet a day for as long as you are on the diet. I prefer to use a vitamin preparation which contains minerals as well just for good measure, because when you tamper with a diet to which you have been accustomed it is very difficult for anybody to know the exact differences you are making in intake of dietary factors other than the basic protein, fat and carbohydrate. There are all sorts of other subtleties including trace elements which are known now to be of importance.

Apart from the fact that any diet may or may not be beneficial to multiple sclerosis I have found that a diet has other advantages. For me it has been a positive course of action and although I know that it is not a definitive cure for multiple sclerosis I do know that I am doing something about it and something that has the blessing of the majority of well-informed doctors. I think that the very fact of being on a regime, and one to which you could adhere strictly, gives you a certain security and feeling of hope. This could be dismissed as ridiculous suggestibility but I believe it has greater significance than this. There is a certain calm which follows the decision to embark on a definitive course of action and remain on that course until there is scientific evidence that it is mistaken. One of the polyunsaturated fatty acids is linoleic acid which is an essential fatty acid. This means that it has to be present in the food eaten because the body is unable to manufacture it. It has been found that the level of linoleic acid in the blood of some patients with multiple sclerosis is reduced and research has been done on the beneficial effects of adding linoleic acid to the diet of patients. So far the published results have not been very conclusive or very encouraging but there does seem to be some evidence that relapses are more rare and of less significance if patients are taking linoleic acid. The linoleic acid is taken in the form of sunflower seed oil or capsules and the amount is directed by the doctor. Again, this addition to the diet can do you no harm and may do some good and many patients, including myself, feel that it is worth trying. The capsules can be bought from health food shops. They are rather expensive but are very much more pleasant to take than the oil. At the time of writing, the capsules are not available on the N.H.S. because they are not of proven value as treatment in multiple sclerosis.

It may be important if you have multiple sclerosis that you lose weight. Obviously, if the muscles in your legs are weak it will not help them to carry around unnecessary pounds. There is also the tendency to take less exercise if you are tired and find it difficult to walk about and you may fail to restrict your food intake to keep pace with your restricted activity. I had a successful slimming campaign when the illness was first diagnosed. I was at that time more than three stone (19kg) overweight possibly due to diminishing activity over the previous years. I lost weight by restricting starch and sugar as well as fats but probably lost it much too fast. A steady weight loss of about one and a half to two pounds (approximately 0·5–1·0kg) a week is ideal. You will have to keep an eye on your weight indefinitely but you may well find, as I have, that once your target weight is achieved you can relax about eating starch and sugar as long as you are on a low fat diet. If you do not allow yourself a reasonable amount of starch and sugar you may be eating insufficient calories and you may lose more weight than is necessary and get tired and listless.

CHAPTER EIGHT

Exercise and Rest

Both exercise and rest seem to me very important parts of learning to live with multiple sclerosis. In the early days and during bad patches I found, and still do find, that having something positive to do and a routine to follow gives me a greater feeling of security and a lot of reassurance; in the same way as accepting and sticking to a diet, so rest and exercise does help. Nobody knows for certain the value of rest or of exercise in multiple sclerosis but there seems little doubt that if both are used as a regular pattern of life then one will be physically fitter even if there is no lasting benefit for multiple sclerosis.

There was a time when complete bed rest for multiple sclerosis was advised in acute phases and relapses. This is probably still practised to some extent but I think many doctors would query the value of remaining in bed for the whole of each twenty-four hours. Weak muscles can get weaker, unpleasant spasms are more likely to occur and balance may be lost. At times of acute fatigue after making a journey or just indulging in too much activity I know from experience that a fair amount of rest for a few days can bring about a quite dramatic improvement. I have never spent a whole day in bed during the time that I have known I had multiple sclerosis. I probably have a rather illogical feeling that as long as I am on the move at sometime during each waking hour of every day I shall put off indefinitely the time at which I should not be able to walk about. Others might benefit from more rest but I should become very anxious if forced to remain bed.

Certainly the principle of a fair amount of rest when the symptoms are troublesome or fatigue is extreme seems sensible. There is a difference between taking one walk around the house every hour to keep oneself mobile, stretch one's legs and keep a better sense of balance, and a lot of pottering around during which tiredness can be made worse and little useful exercise taken. Dr. Swank also recommended that a daily rest in the middle of the day should be taken for an indefinite time by all patients with multiple sclerosis. The rest time should be increased to twice a day during any bad patches. It is surprising that there are so many housewives who have no commitments outside the home who say they are quite unable to find the time for a regular daily rest. Perhaps if they have young children it really is not possible but if something seems important enough it can usually be fitted into a day's routine somehow. A housewife must become as competent at administering her time and energy as a company executive is in running his firm. I am not writing this in any way as a super organiser but because I know that it is possible in nearly all circumstances with a little forward planning and the right emphasis on priorities. It does help if you are not too obsessional about housework! If the time you have planned for your rest arrives and you have not cleared up the lunch I am sure in the long run it is better to leave the chores and have your rest.

Learning to live at a reasonable speed and with sufficient rest and avoiding undue fatigue is an art. I am sure it can more easily be acquired by some people than by others. I am amongst those who find it very difficult to come to terms with recurrent and severe fatigue. If I feel well I forget about a rest and can spend several days feeling well and doing very much more than is reasonable. By the time fatigue has caught up with me I am unable to sleep properly because of spasms in my leg muscles and twitchings and it can take several weeks, when I am forced to limit my activity, before I am functioning reasonably well again. It is very stupid because more of one's life can be used profitably if one learns to ration the amount of activity one undertakes and remembers the need for regular rest. This seems to be a fairly widespread problem among multiple sclerosis patients and perhaps the very nature of the illness makes it more difficult to avoid an 'all go' and an 'all stop' way of living.

Avoiding fatigue is not only important for you but also for your family and friends and for those with whom you work. Fatigue will not only make you feel very discouraged, possibly depressed, and many of your symptoms worse; it will also affect those around you. If you get too tired you will have less energy to cope with family and especially the children's problems. It is strange how in some families life seems to fall apart if one of the parents, possibly more often the mother, is not up to par. You cannot rely on other people to see that you rest enough and do not overwork and overtire yourself. It really is your responsibility to learn how much you can manage without getting tired; it is part of the process of learning to live with multiple sclerosis. The art of managing a rest in the middle of the day unobtrusively, and as often as possible, is a difficult one to learn but I think it is possible. Extra rest before an unusually tiring weekend does seem to give some benefit. If you are working outside the home it is even more difficult to manage a daily rest. Even with part-time work it can be difficult and I know that I have had great difficulty in planning half-time work so that I need only work half of each day. To remain in an optimum state of health and be able to give and to get the maximum pleasure from life it has to be organised somehow.

When you do manage to sit down, make it a habit to put your feet up, lean back and relax. It is a help to have a leg extension for a chair or some sort of chaise longue at hand in a warm and convenient room. Resting your body is helped if you can also rest your mind at the same time. For many lively minded people this is not necessarily achieved by doing nothing. Possibly listening to music will help you to relax, or reading the daily paper or a novel. The worst thing to do is to lie down and let your mind run round the chores that are waiting to be done while you do nothing. There is an art in doing the maximum amount of work with the least effort; a great deal of energy can be used very unprofitably by standing around talking or just pottering about. I keep a stool by the telephone so that I need not waste effort standing while speaking on the telephone; during a long telephone call I slip quietly on to the floor and lie flat on my back and relax. Unfortunately, there is a window by the telephone overlooked by the path to the house but so far nobody has found me prostrate on the floor!

I think yoga could possibly be a good way of exercising and learning to relax at the same time. I find it is not something that I can learn from books or even from watching television programmes—I should need to go to classes and have been tempted to attend some at the time of writing this book. Unfortunately, it means a round trip of fifty miles one evening a week and I feel that the drive, when tired, would do more harm than the yoga would do good. If you have classes near at hand it might be very useful because it could be possible to learn exercise and useful methods of relaxation and rest at the same time.

The whole question of exercise is as beset with difficulties as that of rest. The value of a certain amount of exercise in the management of multiple sclerosis would not be queried by the vast majority of doctors, but the amount of exercise and the type of exercise recommended would vary considerably according to the views of the doctor in charge as well as the severity of the multiple sclerosis. The neurologist who laid most stress on regular exercise and a particular form of exercise is W. Ritchie Russell, formerly Professor of Clinical Neurology at Oxford. He has written a book on his views using records of some of his patients; it is easy reading for the general public. He believes that the course of multiple sclerosis can be influenced by increasing the amount of blood supplied to the brain and improving what he calls the 'blood brain barrier'. He believes also that push-ups are the most effective form of exercise because they improve the circulation, particularly in the upper part of the body, neck and brain. He has worked out a regime which he firmly believes can have a markedly favourable influence not only on the present state of multiple sclerosis, if in a period of relapse, but in the long term outlook also. This regime needs to be followed for an indefinite period of time.

His regime started because he found that handicapped multiple sclerosis patients who were at Stoke Mandeville Hospital and who joined in the programme of exercises for those patients with spinal injuries showed marked improvement. He worked out a scheme of twenty-four hours bed rest in an acute relapse and then a programme of rest and exercise which varied for each patient. This was called the rest exercise programme (R.E.P.). The exercise was usually so many push-ups, varying in number, either followed or preceded by total rest. This programme might be done hourly or twice a day. The book makes fascinating reading, particularly the case histories and anecdotes of the twenty-one patients. I would not attempt to undermine anybody's personal belief in the efficacy of such a programme, but I personally am not impressed by the rather sketchy and inconsistent evidence given by so small a number of patients. I think that the idea of a twice daily period of exercise until slightly sweating followed by a rest is probably a very good one, and there may also be some benefit in increasing the rate of circulation in the head and neck area. I do not find, however, that I get the most benefit from one particular exercise repeated for an indefinite period but rather from different exercises at different times according to the need of the moment. If you are the sort of person who can really be committed to two regular spells of twenty minutes a day, this is probably beneficial. I find that my periods of exercise are erratic in time although I do usually manage two periods each day even though they are not at regular times.

The value of organised physiotherapy on a regular basis is doubtful. For most patients and most physiotherapists, unless the patient is in hospital, a short regular daily session is impossible. Irregular lengthy sessions may be too tiring at the time and not be repeated sufficiently often at home. The ideal seems to be that exercises should be taught as required, or as recommended by the doctor, and these should then be worked on quietly at home on a regular basis. Occasional visits should be made to the physiotherapist for supervision or for working out new exercises. My first exercises were worked out with the aid of my athlete son and were geared to strengthening all my limbs. I found that exercises to stretch the backs of my legs were very difficult at first but could be managed much more easily in a warm bath.

I have found that I have always needed to do exercises to

strengthen my left arm and left leg. I have also had to do regular exercises to help the backs of both legs remain stretched. At times I have had to work hard to stop my left wrist staying flexed forwards; it is an effort to get the wrist bent back and because the hand is clumsy it is easy to stop using it much. Recently I have found it more difficult to keep my head upright and also to sit upright. If I sit for longer than about half an hour my back aches in the upper part. Back and neck strengthening exercises are helping a great deal and I think the most sensible way is to exercise regularly but to concentrate on parts that seem to be in particular need at any one time.

Many people with multiple sclerosis seem to be troubled with muscle spasms and sometimes with muscle twitchings. I have found that the backs of my thighs are liable to go into spasms when sitting on a soft chair or a soft car seat and also in bed at night if I am particularly tired. It is not painful but is an unpleasant feeling and is quite sufficient to stop me sleeping. I have found, by a process of trial and error, that the most effective way of stopping the spasm is by exercising and strengthening the 'antagonists'. The antagonists of a muscle are those that work in the opposite direction; thus if the muscles at the back of the thigh are in spasm, straight leg raising which will make the muscles on the front of the thigh work hard will help the spasm. In a car, where straight leg raising is not feasible, lifting the thigh off the seat while pressing down on the knee gives relief from the spasm.

You may say, if you are a housewife and finding your ordinary chores tiring, that the last thing you require is exercise! In some ways you could be right but in other ways I think you are wrong. Perhaps it would be possible to organise the chores so that they are less exhausting, and delegate the jobs you find most tiring. I have found that it is far less tiring to prepare the evening meal first thing in the morning so that I do not have to cope with it when I come in exhausted in the evening. Housework is not necessarily the best exercise and is not likely to cover all the body movements that need to be used. I think it is far better to organise life to have time for more rest, spend two periods each day doing particular exercises and, in addition, to walk at least a mile a day if possible. I was advised to get a static cycle for use when the weather was too bad for walking. At first I did use it quite frequently because I tended to blow over very easily in the wind in the north of Scotland, but now that I am a little more stable I can walk in most weathers. Now I use the cycle very little, but I can imagine there could be times when I should use it more frequently. Meantime it is used most often for endurance tests by my son and some of his more energetic friends! It seems to be a re-markably robust machine and causes a great deal of delight to other people.

CHAPTER NINE

Friends and Help

'No man is an island'—perhaps this will really strike you forcibly for the first time when you come to face all the problems of living with a chronic and possibly disabling illness such as multiple sclerosis. During the first weeks after the diagnosis is made you may well be too stunned to be much affected by your friends and their help. If you are going to make a good emotional adjustment and live as positively as it is possible to do, you are going to need your friends and their help as never before. Some of us are lucky and have lived in the same place for years and are surrounded by relatives and good, loyal and tried friends. Others of us have moved around a great deal and have never known quite the same security of many years spent among the same people. Yet others of us do not find it easy to make friends, even though we may live for many years near the same people. Perhaps we are shy, or for one reason or another do not find it easy or pleasant to make close social contact with people. For people like that, an illness such as multiple sclerosis can be a far greater problem in the long run because it will become more difficult to accept help and at one time or another you are going to need help. Perhaps you are married but find that you can really feel only close to one person and confide in your husband. This can put a very great burden on your husband who has his own life to lead and work to do and it can put an unbearable strain on your marriage.

As a doctor, I was much more used to giving help than receiving it and I did find it difficult after the diagnosis was made to realise that I should need help. For me, the need for help was brought home very forcibly because I could not drive or walk as far as a shop or a bus and I had a family to feed. If it had not been for that basic fact of life—hunger—I might have been a lot longer in realising that most people at some time in their lives need to become receivers of help and not givers of help. Having learned to accept offers of help in getting food, and later, when I could walk better, accepting a lift to the nearest town to do my own shopping, it became easier to reconcile myself to accepting other sorts of help.

It could be looked on as commendably courageous and independent to refuse help but I think it is nothing short of selfish. It is one thing to do the things of which you are capable and always be prepared to add to your skills, but to reject offers of help to do those things which you are unable to do, is hurtful for the helper and harmful for yourself. Your relatives and friends know that you are not able to undertake all the things with which you used to cope and if you attempt it you become unduly fatigued. They are not going to go on offering help indefinitely if it is always refused, and if family offers of help are met with curt refusals and irritability, it is not fair to blame them when you get overtired. All of us who are independent by nature hate to admit that we can no longer do everything for ourselves and we are very foolish if we do not come to terms with this fundamental change in our lives early in the illness. If we do not, we shall make our lives very much more difficult for ourselves, more difficult for those we love and those who love us, and as a result will precipitate family unrest and anxiety. Martyrdom is not an attractive characteristic; it is so much better to swallow your pride and accept help with gratitude. Both you and the helper will feel a lot better and as you need more help it will make it easier to ask for it. Friends do not know by instinct the best ways in which they can help you but are usually very willing to be told.

If you are open about the diagnosis of multiple sclerosis from the time you are told, I think that it helps you to accept help. I know that some people prefer to keep such things to themselves, or share it with only their very closest friends. For them this may be right but I have had letters from those who at first kept the illness a secret and later when the symptoms were difficult to hide and they badly needed help could not bring themselves to speak to friends or neighbours and found themselves becoming depressed recluses. I decided early on in the illness that I had to be open about it and it was better that way for all concerned. We live in a village and curiosity is a natural part of village life! You can either look on it as an uninvited and unwelcome invasion of your privacy or you can look on it as I do, as a very natural interest in what is happening to other people in the same small community. Whether my view is right or wrong, I have never had cause to regret my openness about the illness. If you try to keep an illness secret when the doctor is driving frequently to your house and you are no longer appearing around the village, rumour is bound to spread. In our part of the world, if I had not said I had multiple sclerosis, I should long ago have been labelled as an alcoholic. If anybody saw me out now, in the dark or in a high wind, the diagnosis of being an alcoholic would seem even more credible! My honesty was repaid with many kindnesses and a very great deal of encouragement. Even so rumours abounded: I had been at home about a week before I happened to be near the front door when our postman arrived at lunch time with our mail. He looked overjoyed at seeing me up and dressed because he had heard in the village that I was in my bed and would not be getting up again. When I started walking rather slowly up to the village shop, again I was greeted by many people whom I did not know and was much encouraged by their welcome and obvious pleasure in my improvement.

The arrival of the mail became a very vital and eagerly anticipated event in my day. I have never before had so many letters and most of them were enormously helpful. The only letters I learned to dread were the ones saying that the writer had looked the disease up in the *Encyclopaedia Britannica* or elsewhere and was completely horrified that this could have happened to me. This sort of sympathy, if it can be called that, is worse than bad. It is destructive of morale but I learned to harden myself to it and to write a deliberately constructive and optimistic answer to such a letter.

My mother is a very diligent letter writer and I know from her that many of our more distant relatives were doubtful about writing to me because they felt they were out of touch; she encouraged them to write and I am glad that she did. It gave me a great feeling of support to sense the nearness and thought of those, many of whom I had not seen or heard of for many years. It felt good to be in touch again and to hear their news and renew their acquaintance. We have many friends in different parts of the world and it was particularly good to hear from those good friends 'down under'. The world seemed smaller and I did not feel so isolated when reading about friends and their lives in Brisbane, Sydney, or Melbourne. It was up to me to respond to their encouragement and their news and for many weeks, answering their letters was one of my regular daily activities. It became a very favourite activity and I have many regrets that since I started working again, and coping with the resulting fatigue, my letter writing has been allowed to lapse to so great an extent. If you can manage to be a regular letter writer you will never lose good friends however far away they may live. It is in times of illness and isolation that perhaps one really appreciates friends as at no other time. Friendships cannot just be kept for when you are in need. One has to find time to help keep friendships in repair when the going is happier.

It was particularly encouraging to hear about other people with multiple sclerosis who had done very well, and how much their determination seemed to help. I do not know if determination is effective but it certainly spurred me on to do everything I could to help myself. A writer friend suggested that I should keep a detailed diary because being a patient, a medical practitioner and a journalist it might be of use later in my medicine or writing work. It has certainly helped me a lot to keep that diary and once I had written down a problem it often seemed more manageable. I am afraid the diary was kept very much more regularly in the bad times than in the good and I have still not had the courage to read it all. Some of it seems too recent and too painful to be read. I can remember as much as I want to, without reading things written down during the dark times.

I found that the telephone was a mixed blessing. Most phone calls were marvellous and very welcome and cheering. Sometimes there would be an offer to do my shopping or an invitation out for a drive or a trip to town, or later out to coffee or a meal. One of my earliest outings was to our one and only supermarket. After a devastating start with a trolley that went only in circles, I found a more dependable support. The effort of pushing that trolley was such that when I came to pay by cheque at the cash out point I was unable to write. Luckily the cashier knew me and accepted a squiggle. I found that too often I was at the mercy of the person at the other end of the telephone. I learned to dread 'you poor, poor thing, I can't think how you are ever going to manage'. I usually ended up, with such a caller, sorting out her problems rather than receiving help from her with mine! Of course most calls were very welcome and cheerful and often arrived at a time when I was feeling low. I had my favourite callers who somehow always seemed to phone at just the right moment and have just the right sort of thing to say. I found on several occasions that one of the ever-present problems of the telephone is that you cannot read it again at leisure and have another think about it. The sound has disappeared and much as you would like to hear a word or a phrase again it has gone. Apart from calls from some friends I have found that letters are far more comforting and enduring than telephone calls. Sometimes I would read and re-read them and they never left me with the rather lost feeling that a telephone call might. Perhaps at a time of shock and insecurity the physical presence of paper and writing is one of greater comfort and help than the ephemeral nature of another voice however pleasant at the time. I would excuse one special call from that generalisation. It was a special piece of help that came from a friend and I shall never forget it. It was during my first week at home and she phoned and said casually that there was a phone by her bed and if I ever felt like a chat during the night she would be there. That meant a great deal to me at the time and probably far more than she will ever know.

I found visitors a great delight. I much preferred somebody to drop in than be asked beforehand if it would be convenient. This is probably a personal idiosyncrasy but I found that my fatigue was so unpredictable that I felt very upset if I was expecting somebody and then felt too tired to be cheerful, whereas if the caller was unexpected it did not seem so shocking to admit that I was very tired. Loans of magazines and novels gave me great pleasure. I had seldom before in my adult life had so much leisure time in which to read and although I always have books waiting to be read, other people's favourites were very welcome additions.

It is important to acquire the habit and never lose it, of taking as much interest in your friends and their affairs as they are good enough to be taking in yours. You have the time when you are not well to listen to other people's problems; think how they can best be helped, and perhaps have time for discussions which may be useful. Learning to live with illness includes learning to use your own problems constructively in order to be outgoing and helpful to others. Self-centredness and self-pity will bring you nothing but regrets, isolation and depression. You must try from the beginning to look outwards rather than inwards and learn to meet other people in their world rather than trying to bring them into yours; this is particularly so if at the time you may not be finding yours an especially happy one. Learn to listen; get to know people better; find out what makes them happy and try to understand their problems. Theirs may be far greater than yours although they have not got a medical name for them and they may have learned a great deal about how to cope with problems which could be helpful to you.

All the help your friends give you, whether it is letters, calls, lifts in cars or just chats on the phone help to make you feel a person. We have talked before about the dangers of feeling a non-person when you know you have a potentially disabling illness where feelings about yourself can change in a subtly negative way. Perhaps the best thing that your friends can do to help are to make you realise that you are still the same 'you', with the same sense of humour, the same spots, the same love of sausages or what-have-you. There are times when this sort of thing, if taken for granted, can be the most useful sort of helping and restoring process.

CHAPTER TEN

Getting Through the Bad Patches

Multiple sclerosis by its very nature is unpredictable and there cannot be many people with it who do not have to come to terms with the bad patches. I find this unpredictability the most difficult thing about learning to live with multiple sclerosis. There are times when I might say with some honesty that I have come to terms with my present problems and can manage my daily life with certain restrictions. Then suddenly a bad patch turns up and I find all my resignation, good intentions and adaptability turned upside down and these are times when I feel I just have to start again from the beginning. The very unexpectedness of these patches makes them more upsetting and much more frightening.

Those with multiple sclerosis find these bad patches among their most distressing times. One woman described herself as quite different when she was exhausted and no longer the woman her husband had married. She said she felt so different during one of these patches when she could be a fiend to her family. She was no longer able to apologise when it was over, for she realised she was not responsible for her behaviour and knew quite certainly that it would happen again. I will talk more about multiple sclerosis and mental effects in Chapter Twelve.

The bad patches need not be as troublesome as this but their occurrence seems inevitable. I used to believe that they were entirely unpredictable or else I blamed a non-existent menopause or anything else of which I could think. I have now come to realise that the bad patches of fatigue, which may or may not be accompanied by other physical problems becoming worse, are to a certain extent predictable. It is possible that there are times when one is more vulnerable to fatigue; perhaps these are when the disease is more active, but there are other times when one's own actions precipitate a bad patch or when family situations or emotional crises precipitate a rough period.

A bad patch can vary in both length and severity. It can be a few days of excessive fatigue when it is very difficult to get through your usual work. Sometimes during these phases of fatigue it is difficult to remain patient and good tempered and it is very distressing to get worried and even angry over things at home with which, at other times, you know perfectly well you could cope. Other bad patches may last longer and as well as fatigue there may be the recurrence or increase of old physical symptoms. This does not necessarily seem to mean that the disease has become active again. There does not seem to be any good explanation for this variability in symptoms from day to day, week to week or even from hour to hour. After the bad patch has passed the chances are that the symptoms will clear up again, a weak leg will be less weak, difficult speech will be less difficult, uncomfortable muscle spasms in your legs may go, and blurred vision will to a certain extent improve again.

Sometimes a bad patch can be a relapse in the disease when new symptoms may occur or old symptoms may get worse and recovery be less complete. A serious relapse must be managed and treated as an acute episode in the illness and medical help will be necessary. Serious relapses are not nearly as frequent as the recurrent bad patches and it is the bad patches rather than serious relapses that I am going to talk about.

It would be a great advantage to patients with multiple sclerosis if there was some clear-cut method of avoiding bad patches. There are probably fairly good ways of preventing many of them, but nobody can give good clear instructions about what to do and what not to do for any particular individual. There is so much variety and I think the only effective ways of preventing these patches are by coming to know yourself, your own health and your own powers of stamina and signs of fatigue. It all sounds so simple but I do not think that

I am alone in finding this art one of the most difficult to acquire in living with multiple sclerosis. If you are feeling well you will naturally want to forget about having anything wrong with you. Possibly you also have the urge to cram in all you possibly can while you are feeling well. I know that I do both of these things and am only slowly and painfully learning to live with more moderation. Possibly the biggest incentive for me to try and learn to live at a more moderate pace is that in the end I achieve more of what I want to do if I can carry on at a snail's pace than keep having to stop if I do spurts like a hare and then have weeks when I can do very little indeed.

There are some ways of coming to terms with work and life that make bad patches less likely and more easily controlled. In medical terms primary prevention is to avoid the thing ever starting and secondary prevention is to catch it early and treat it vigorously. In one way primary prevention is not possible in multiple sclerosis because the multiple sclerosis lesion is there and the vulnerability to fatigue is always present. It is really early secondary prevention that we are talking about; the things that we can do or not do to prevent bad patches and the most effective ways of coping with them if and when they do occur.

Many people with multiple sclerosis find that they have long spells when they really do seem to have far more energy, and are less prone to fatigue and at times like these it is normal and natural to forget about the illness and get on with life and all its opportunities. Some people now may remain on a non-animal fat or other diet however well they are but others will carry on with their lives without any controls or restrictions. They may get away with it for many years and there is nothing to say that they would have been better or postponed a relapse longer if they had kept to some sort of regime. Other people have phases of being very much more vulnerable to fatigue, either over a limited time or over many years. I think that for people who have to cope with this problem on a more or less permanent basis and who naturally want to lead as full a life as possible, there are one or two possibilities that may make the smooth periods more on a level with the rough periods. I do think that although many rough periods seem to be completely un-

77

predictable there are perhaps a few ways of trying to avoid them.

Any fatigue is bad and exhaustion is really bad, therefore fatigue and exhaustion should be avoided. It is difficult for many of us to ration our activity and particularly our output of emotional energy but that is just what we are going to have to learn. I find that one late night a week is as much as I can manage. I used to be able to have several late nights in a row and have a good sleep at the weekend, and feel quite refreshed and carry on the next week full of energy. Now I am best with no late nights but an occasional one is virtually unavoidable. I have to ration myself and make polite excuses for the meetings and social occasions that I know I shall not be able to manage. The greatest risk is when I feel fittest and am sure that I can manage three late nights in a row. After the first I begin to wilt and am much more tired the second evening. I am very grateful if I am gently bullied by one of the family into phoning and making my apologies for the third event. I know that for many, as for me, it goes against the grain to fail to do those things that one has undertaken; priorities must always be kept in the right order. From being one who regularly burnt the midnight oil I find that I am now far better if I am in bed by 10 p.m. or earlier, as often as I am able. If I know that I have a heavy working day or any other particularly strenuous day ahead of me I go to bed even earlier. Sometimes it is difficult and even embarrassing to arrange this but for me it is worth it and I know of others who find that it is worthwhile. It is said that you are unable to store sleep like charging a battery but from my experience it is quite possible to save energy by more rest and more sleep before undertaking anything that I know will be particularly tiring.

Many people with multiple sclerosis find that travelling, and particularly long journeys in cars, is very tiring. On a very small scale we have had the comfort of the front seats of our car improved for me by having them re-upholstered more firmly. Even so, I do find long car journeys exhausting. I used to enjoy travelling very much and was too interested to be tired. Now, however, I think very hard before making any journey. I have a feeling that a considerable number of multiple sclerosis relapses follow holidays. Possibly the best sort of holiday for the person with multiple sclerosis is one at home with even the thought of exporting all or part of the rest of the family! I find that if I have to travel a long distance within the United Kingdom a night sleeper is the least tiring way of doing it and not by air. Even a short Continental journey I find less tiring by train and a night crossing by boat but I still take several days to recover from such a journey. I have a feeling that a lengthy trip in a cargo boat in a cool climate might be the ideal holiday but I have yet to see the opportunity of putting this dream into practice!

Getting overheated at any time is liable to precipitate fatigue and make symptoms worse. I find that having been a sun worshipper for most of my life I can no longer tolerate the sun. I sometimes sit out in a sheltered spot in October or November in the north of Scotland but even at that latitude I am unable to sit in the sun in the summer months. If I do, all my symptoms are worse and my feeling of exhaustion can be very great; I have even found that a hot bath and an electric blanket are unhelpful. I have not gone as far as self-inflicted chilling but sometimes I am aware that I feel so much better in cool weather that I am tempted to strip off some of my clothing and try just a minimum amount of covering.

To avoid bad patches a counsel of perfection is to lead as peaceful and well organised a life as possible. To start with the most simple things, I have made great efforts to be more tidy so that I know where all my possessions are and can find anything with the minimum of effort. The system falls down when somebody walks off with my kitchen scissors and uses them for cutting their nails in the bathroom. Incredible but true! It is very much more difficult to learn to live a relaxed life without emotional upsets especially if you happen to have a houseful of children of any ages but perhaps particularly teenagers. Probably any type of mental organisation, from Christian discipline to transcendental meditation may help. I am no expert on either but I feel sure that a daily routine of mental rest and relaxation as well as physical exercise and diet will give a more balanced way of living.

If, or much more probably, when, you run into a bad patch

while taking every precaution and often through circumstances which you do not understand or over which you have no control, I can only suggest some methods that may be helpful. If you are able to 'switch off' and abandon daily chores for a short while it is much better. It may be best to stay with a good friend for a day or two if it is difficult to get real rest at home. I know one lovely quiet country inn, not too far away, where I am always welcome and I find the sort of peace, hospitality and indeed spoiling which in itself is healing. In a matter of hours my fatigue begins to lift; I sometimes wish I had the time and money to go there for a regular long weekend every month.

Perhaps if your children are older you will be able to have a few days in bed now and again when you are very tired. I try to keep a plentiful supply of food in the house, both dried and in the freezer, to cater for such times. My own family are very good and will cope with house and animals while I have a day in bed at a weekend when I am very tired. I find that if I am going through a more prolonged bad spell (so far I have managed without taking any time off work), I can help myself a little by staying longer in bed in the morning if I do not have to be at work early. I also have a small immersion heater by my bed which is a great blessing for making hot drinks. In bad patches I go to bed very early, perhaps half past seven in the evening and try never to miss my afternoon rest.

I think it is especially important to keep to a disciplined way of life through bad patches. It is much easier for me to write this than stick to it myself! It is so easy to feel that one may as well cheat with your diet, perhaps let yourself put on a bit too much weight, not bother about exercises because you feel too tired. None of these things in themselves may make a lot of difference but the negative attitude of not caring is self-destructive and not helpful to speeding recovery.

It is quite an art to get enough rest and yet not lose touch with friends and interests and so hibernate. You may need to write more letters, use the telephone more (avoiding the high charge times), and make the effort when you do get out to pop in and see somebody you have been meaning to look up even if it is only to leave a few flowers or a magazine. It is very difficult to remain outward looking when literally shut in your house with your own fatigue and sometimes unhappy preoccupations.

Above all it is important never to give up hope however bad the patch is or however long it lasts. I do know how impossible it is at times to keep even a glimmer of hope but very surprising things can and do happen. Sometimes they are very small things; but as long as hope remains alive a very small thing, perhaps just a smile or a word, can mean a very great deal.

CHAPTER ELEVEN

Multiple Sclerosis
and the Family

The diagnosis of multiple sclerosis for the mother or father of a family must have some impact on the family whether it is realised and faced or not. A diagnosis of this sort with all its uncertainties and possible developments cannot leave a family unchanged. If the development of the multiple sclerosis is more rapid and disabling the future stability of the family is more at risk. I have seen one such family where the mother took to a wheelchair against medical advice, at a comparatively early stage of the disease because she felt tired. Her husband has given up his work and now lives at home to look after his wife and their small son. The small son is becoming difficult to control and I have the feeling he uses either parent as a pawn in his own self-seeking. He is too young to understand the illness but he is quite old enough to understand his own powers of manipulation in a difficult and unhappy situation.

I think multiple sclerosis in a parent or in an elder offspring is and should be a family affair. It is not like a cold that will get better or a broken leg that will mend but it is likely to be a long drawn out illness with good times and bad times and always with uncertainty. Such a situation cannot be faced by one member of a family in isolation while the others go on their own way unknowing or uncaring. At least they can, and sometimes they do, but it is a loss of enormous significance both to the member with multiple sclerosis and for the rest of the family. For the marriage, an illness such as multiple sclerosis in one of the partners can be a force leading either to its strengthening or to its disruption.

It is bound to make a big difference whether the patient with multiple sclerosis is the mother or father of the family and also at what stage of disablement the diagnosis is made. If the father is a dentist and his hands are affected he will have to change his occupation. Changing an occupation for anybody, especially a man, is a profoundly disturbing experience. It will probably be more difficult if the patient is older and also more difficult in times of unemployment. The Disablement Resettlement Officer (D.R.O.) may be of some use and this is discussed further in Chapter Seventeen on statutory help. It is probably a mistake to take a decision about change of employment too rapidly. Multiple sclerosis is at all times an unpredictable illness and a good and lengthy remission may occur unexpectedly. If a former employer of a patient can wait and keep his old job open for him or even be prepared to give him part-time or less arduous work to do, it will probably be far more beneficial for both the patient and his family. Knowing that there is work ahead is an enormous comfort and an incentive to do all within one's powers to get better. Perhaps if one did not enjoy working the situation would be different.

A mother or wife with multiple sclerosis will be less likely to be in regular employment. If a father is unable to return to an ordinary job it will be far better for him and his family if he can be out part of the day in some form of sheltered occupation even if his wife starts to work to help with the family income. Many men who are around the house all day not only feel in the way but often are in the way! They are bored and can too easily pass the time with cigarettes, alcohol and television.

A mother or wife with multiple sclerosis will probably not be the sole bread-winner for the family and she may feel less tired if she gives up her part-time work outside her home. If she has children still at home of whatever age she will probably find that she has plenty to do to use her limited energy. She will need more help in the house with certain chores long before anybody need think about adapting the house for a wheelchair or other walking aid.

I was already living many hundreds of miles away from my husband when the diagnosis was made and my initial reaction was to tell neither my husband nor my children. I probably did not want to tell my husband because previous illnesses had been put down to 'all in the mind' and with this sort of illness I think he has little sympathy. Instinctively I shied away from being told once again that I should be all right if I could learn to pull myself together. Eventually I told him and the initial reaction was as I had predicted. When he finally came north our general practitioner saw him and tried to explain but there was a disturbing rift between us. Probably he did care and was unable to show it. Perhaps he was frightened and could not let me know. I think he also found it very difficult to accept that any part of him—even his wife—had an illness which could not be put right. He is a perfectionist and perhaps being faced with an incurable illness was too much for him to take without being damaged himself. He preferred to escape from the situation in intense work in the south. Looking back at it now I can be philosophical but at the time I was far more aware of my own sense of rejection and loss. It was a very unhappy feeling to be permanently down-graded to a second and for this reason be unwanted. I desperately needed his help and support but I could not travel south and he was too busy to travel north. I think the telephone is the worst possible form of communication at such times. I tried to write letters but they could not be honest or my horrific self-pity showed through them. I felt very rejected and cast aside. These feelings may have been unbalanced but at the time they were too vivid, and too real, and the effort to keep them covered too great to worry about how they matched up with reality. Probably on the surface I appeared calm and under control but at times my feelings of hurt and despair were almost intolerable. I had probably never before needed the closeness and support of a loving husband as much as I did at that time and I did not even have the physical presence of my husband.

Ironically on the rare occasions when he did come north I tried so hard to cover up my hurt feelings that I probably seemed to him hard and unloving and rejecting. Those weekends were invariably the ones when there were children in the house, that I was particularly tired and always ended in bickering and an increased gap between us. I think that these feelings were the hardest I had to bear and perhaps, who knows, my husband was suffering as much but in a different way. Looking back it is easy to be wise and see what might have happened if one had behaved differently. Over the past year the situation has improved a great deal and my husband says this is because I seem different. I am not able to explain to him that of course I do seem different now that I am not treated as a reject model or a leper. It is probably better to let such feeling drift and be patient and receptive to change and improvement and keep hoping.

I think and I have also noticed when any chronic or severe illness affects one member of a married couple the result can either be a bonding process or a disrupting one. Probably this depends on the maturity of the characters involved and the depth of mutual regard and affection which they can bring to, and share in dealing with, the problem. False courage, bravado, sympathy, and demanding behaviour and childish ways all tend to disrupt the relationship. In our particular instance sheer physical distance between us, the impossibility of spending much time together and probably my own over-defensiveness all combined to act as disruptive factors. In a close marriage it is impossible to hide deep feelings, fears of disability, fears of death and fears for the future. If they can be shared, much emotional isolation can be avoided and there is a much greater chance that the marriage will be strengthened rather than weakened.

Open discussion may be needed about money, for when either a husband or wife is disabled, the amount of effective money for the use of the family inevitably drops. If the husband is unable to work, a disability pension, possibly other insurances, and savings are unlikely to be as great as his original income. The wife may not be able to go out to work for many hours a day to supplement the family income because she may be needed at home to help her husband, and cope with the daily chores. If the wife is disabled through multiple sclerosis she will be entitled to the disability pension and possibly the attendance allowance as well as the new non-contributory invalidity pension for married women. It is very unlikely that these financial aids will really recompense the family for the extra expense incurred in replacing the lost work of a wife and mother. Help will be needed for cooking, cleaning and possibly caring for children as well as for the disabled mother. In addition the husband may find that he has to refuse promotion or to take time off work to cope with many everyday problems with which his wife would normally have dealt.

Then there is the question of children. Should children be told about a sick parent, and if they are told how much should they be told and when? It is very difficult to generalise with such a complicated problem. Very small children may be unaware of the family difficulties as long as their physical and emotional needs are attended to by an effective mother substitute. At any age older than this I think there is a far greater danger in under- rather than over-estimating the understanding of children. If they are not told about an illness such as multiple sclerosis their suffering and their sense of exclusion may be much greater than if they are told gently and progressively kept informed about the illness. It is all important that their questions should be answered honestly and as fully as they require to be. Obviously this needs a subtlety of judgement which many parents may lack. It is probably more difficult to tell adolescent children than to tell younger children. Adolescence is a very vulnerable time when feelings both positive and negative may be running high between parents and offspring. I think there are few homes where they can honestly say that there are not occasional emotional crises during these years. What is going to be the effect on an adolescent of being told that a parent has a progressive and incurable illness such as multiple sclerosis?

I think the same sort of approach should be used in telling the adolescent as in telling the patient. Honesty is paramount but optimism comes a close second. Multiple sclerosis is not a death sentence; rather it is a diagnosis that needs some thought and considerable adaptation of life style. If this can be sensibly explained to an adolescent then the fact of excessive fatigue on the part of the mother or father and the consequent demands on him/her to give help will not be such a problem.

My own three adolescents were told formally by our general

practitioner when I was brought back from the hospital after I had crashed my car. I did not hear what he said because I was in bed and they were in the kitchen. They asked me no questions and made no comments and I was foolish enough to take this to mean that they had taken in the situation and accepted it. How could any doctor whom they did not know particularly well, have made such good contact with them in a matter of minutes? Probably because we are effectively a one-parent family we normally discuss anything and everything at some length but on this occasion I kept my thoughts and feelings to myself. I suppose if I had been asked why I did so I should have answered that I felt that the children had had enough to put up with, such as the drastic change of schooling and of culture and the vulnerability of a one-parent family, to have to face the problems of their mother's health. I thought innocently that as long as I was around the house, got their breakfast for them before they went to school and had a meal ready for them when they came in that was enough.

I was so very wrong and did not see that my reticence was not sparing their feelings but making the situation far more tense and their suffering greater. I was on my diet and taking sunflower seed oil but I did not comment on it. It irritated the children's already jagged nerves, and my son went to a trusted friend of ours and said how impossible the situation at home was becoming and how completely obsessed I was with my illness and everything to do with it. I think this was an example of words left unsaid speaking louder than words that are said. I was bitterly ashamed of myself and of the way in which I had let my children down while proudly believing I had been doing and saying the best things for them. How wrong and misguided we can be even when we believe we have the best intentions. I tried to put matters right but do not think I was very intelligent about that either.

One evening I was more than usually tired and down; after I had given the children their meal I went and lay down on my bed and cried. After a little while my eldest came and sat down beside me. She took my arm and gently ticked me off. She told me they all knew I had multiple sclerosis and they had found out a lot about it. They respected me for trying to keep it to myself but it was wrong of me because I should have realised that they were not small children but people who were quite old enough to help me and share my problems. Whatever the future holds for her or for me or for both of us I shall always remember that moment with profound gratitude for her understanding and wisdom.

Is it wrong that children or young people should be forced into situations like this before one believes they are ready to face the harder facts of life? Obviously it must depend on the young people themselves, the family as a whole and the strength of the individual bond within the family. Of course they forget, are careless, thoughtless and occasionally utterly callous but that is how it should be. Yet underneath the natural behaviour of adolescents towards their middle-aged parents I know that mine have an unusual protectiveness which may only be shown by a push away from the kitchen sink and an instruction to go and have an early bath and not take all the hot water.

It is as necessary for a parent with multiple sclerosis to be optimistic with her children as it is necessary for a doctor to be optimistic with his patients. There is no point in pondering about an unhappy future and it is much more important to concentrate on the possibilities of today. It is also very important that a parent should at no time blackmail children with her illness. I know from bitter personal experience that this can all too easily happen and at the time be done unwittingly. You must be extremely honest with yourself about your motives and never let personal gain, through your disability or potential disability, influence your actions or your attitude towards your family.

CHAPTER TWELVE

Multiple Sclerosis
and its Mental Effects

Multiple sclerosis is known as a physical disease which affects nervous tissue and not as a mental disease. There are many medical phrases used in connection with multiple sclerosis such as 'psychological overlay' when describing symptoms, the 'M.S. personality' and 'M.S. euphoria'. These do suggest that doctors realise that multiple sclerosis does have well observed mental effects. There is the frequency of misdiagnosis of multiple sclerosis as a psychiatric illness and there is also the medical impression that emotional problems cannot only be the results of multiple sclerosis but also the cause of relapses. I have talked about many of these ideas elsewhere in this book but I think they are of such importance to many people with multiple sclerosis that I am going to collect some of them together in this chapter and add some new ideas.

Multiple sclerosis and its related mental effects are so closely tied up together and it is known that physical damage is done to nerve tissue in the brain that sometimes I wonder if some of the more distressing mental effects of multiple sclerosis are not just medical or patients' concepts but are actually due to damage to the brain. At times if you are going through a particularly trying period of fatigue and depression it might be a help and a comfort to be able to blame it on physical damage to your brain. It would at least absolve you from some of the responsibility and feelings of guilt that go with moods and behaviour which are trying, to say the least of it, for your family, and provoke a great deal of anxiety in yourself. At other times the very thought that you might have some irreversible physical damage to your brain is quite horrifying. The demyelination can show up on an electroencephalogram so that it obviously could be quite widespread, and remarkably little seems to be known about the physical effects of the scattered demyelination. Multiple sclerosis as a crippling disease is the fact that everybody know about. Multiple sclerosis with deeply distressing mental effects is a disease about which little seems to be known and no sources of knowledge are available to which upset patients can turn for information and help.

Many neurologists have little doubt that emotional upsets can cause actual physical damage in multiple sclerosis, as well as worsening of symptoms which may or may not be due to actual physical damage in the nervous system. During an illness such as multiple sclerosis there is no doubt that you are more likely to have emotional upsets than when you are in good health. There are difficulties with fatigue, with adjustment in learning to do less, there are frequent family difficulties when Mum is less capable of doing her usual share and there is always a certain measure, variable indeed but recurrent, of personal anxiety. Whether one thinks about it consciously or not there is some apprehension about the future, about decreasing mobility and for some people a real fear of losing their independence.

Avoiding emotional upsets and tensions is one of the most difficult parts of living with multiple sclerosis. I think one has to be very clear-headed and almost brutal in facing the situations which are likely to cause emotional problems, preventing them if possible and minimising them if they cannot be prevented. For everybody the situations are bound to be different and of course the solutions must also be different. For everybody the same amount of honesty is necessary in facing up to the situations and the same sort of determination in finding possible solutions. Fatigue is probably the most important factor in exacerbating emotional problems. It is very much easier to be philosophical about marital problems, difficult situations at work, adolescent offsprings' love problems and unexpected visitors, if one is not already overtired.

I have found that with a little clear thinking I have been able to do a few things towards reducing the situations that cause fatigue. I find car driving very tiring and because I have to drive long distances possibly get more tired by the anticipation that fatigue is inevitable. I decided if I could keep my mind off fatigue it might help and my son obligingly installed an inexpensive stereo-cassette player in my car one weekend. It may not work for everybody but I find that if I can have gentle favourite music in the background when I am tired I am very much less aware of my fatigue. I now have the additional support of my son's co-driving. Few mothers with cars have been so keen for their sons to be able to drive them! Whether it is all in the mind or not, that small problem of fatigue has been relieved a little. The only problem arises when I have one of my teenagers with me and have to suffer punk rock instead of floating blissfully through Beethoven's Choral Symphony. However, one must not become intolerant and possibly in time my tastes will broaden!

It is said that euphoria or undue cheerfulness occurs in multiple sclerosis but I have not seen it or experienced it and I think depression is very much more common. Depression can occur at many stages of the disease. It seems to be common in the early stages after the diagnosis is made and the full implication gradually sinks in. I know personally it can be brought on transiently by seeing advertisements for wheelchairs at a time when the real meaning of multiple sclerosis is beginning to be understood. After a good period followed by worsening of symptoms, a bad attack of fatigue or a more serious relapse, patients are very likely to feel depression. These feelings of depression can be severe and very distressing and they do in some people lead to suicide. Some doctors treat such periods of depression with anti-depressants as they would a normal depressive illness. Possibly this is the right treatment but perhaps it overlooks the real cause of the depression. I have been given anti-depressants but have found them of little or no value. On the other hand explanation, reassurance, encouragement, and insistence on physical rest have relieved my depression very effectively. Now that I know that depression does occur I can treat it quickly and effectively myself by getting more physical rest. I do not think it is like an ordinary depressive illness because I find that as soon as I am flat and relaxed I have no difficulty at all in concentrating on a book or writing.

I think it is very important that one should learn to come to terms with these times of depression because they are very unnerving and distressing. They do seem to be a part of the illness of multiple sclerosis in a great number of people. If they can be accepted as an inevitable part of the illness and usually associated with fatigue they need not be felt as so overwhelming. If they are not accepted, I think they can cause very real feelings of guilt at being unable to control one's feelings, cause irritability and lead to fears that one's mind is being permanently affected. They come but they pass and they are something that have to be avoided as far as possible but when unavoidable accepted philosophically. So easy to write, so difficult to do!

Even minor disability has its mental effects. A dragging leg, a weak hand, a clumsy grasp and so on can be very much more obvious to the patient than to the onlooker. If you cannot accept these things as part of yourself and realise that they in no way change the essential you it is possible to become very sensitive about them and even aggressive. Let people help you; it is much more attractive to let somebody else pour out the coffee than upset the coffee pot. People are glad to help and may even feel hurt and rejected themselves if you refuse help. I have said this before but I think it is very important. Life will be much more harmonious for you, your family and your friends if you are able to face the things which you are not able to manage, stop trying to cover up your disability and accept the help that is waiting to be given.

I suppose we all know those magnificent lines of Wordsworth:

> 'Getting and spending we lay waste our powers,
> Little we see in nature that is ours,
> We have given our hearts away, a sordid boon.'

Perhaps they only hit some of us with their full meaning when our powers are lessened and the trivialities of all the getting and spending in our lives is only too apparent. Cut down on some of the mad doings and rushing and acquiring and allow your-self the leisure to stand and stare. I am sure that only in this way can we hope to keep our minds at peace and to have the reserves of strength to deal with the really important things which for so many of us involve ourselves and our families.

Feeling ashamed of our failures and disabilities and weak-nesses is a very negative emotion. When I am very tired I lose my balance easily whether I have had one sherry or not. I am appalled by the thought that people will think I am drunk. Is it so really important what 'people' think and is it really worth wasting my mental anxiety on casual observers? My friends know that it happens and know that I drink very little and will help me when I find it difficult to walk because I am giddy. They exhort me to get less tired and I do try and take notice. It is so important not to waste mental regret and embarrassment on incidents that are really so trivial.

It is particularly important that the mother of a family should come to terms with the many emotional problems involved in multiple sclerosis. It is a strange thing that although the father of the family is usually the bread-winner and often the chief physical provider it is the mother who holds the family together as an integrated and, one hopes, loving unit. If her health fails, and probably her mental health is more important than her physical health in this respect, the family can all too easily fall apart. Children can become difficult at home and at school, adolescents may make unfortunate attachments to those of the opposite sex and become involved in drinking and petty delinquency. It seems so unfair to blame these mishaps on a sick mother but she is so often the pivot around which the children gravitate for their emotional and mental security. If she is too preoccupied with her own problems she is naturally quite unable to help her adolescent children with theirs, and all too easily the family unit can disintegrate.

How can she manage her own problems so that she still has the mental energy and the mental calm to cope with the hun-dreds of demands of a growing family? There are crises at ex-amination times, upsets over love affairs, even fears of preg-nancy, and it is not just that you feel guilty that it could be your fault—in one sense it is your fault, because you are no longer providing the calm and steadying security to which they have been accustomed. They know you are ill, they know you get irritable when you are burdened with problems, they know you get tired with just the minimum amount of work, they try to manage on their own and perhaps take on responsibilities which are beyond their years. They fail and when things which have been hidden come out into the open you realise with some justification that you really have failed them.

There is no question of fault about getting ill but you do have some responsibility for getting tired, irritable, depressed and exhausted. There is the question of responsibility; are you trying to allocate your limited energy in the most sensible way? You must rest during the day. You must stop a job before you are exhausted. If it is possible and certainly, if it is too tiring for you, you must give up a job outside the home. If you do this, remember to fill the vacuum with interests other than your family or you may become even more irritable from boredom than from exhaustion. Do not be afraid to ask for help as cheerfully as you can and accept it sincerely and graciously.

I find that it does help my peace of mind if I try to remember each day, however briefly, the things for which I have to be thankful. This may sound very trite but life can be hard at times and if I can only find ten seconds to remember something for which I am thankful I hope that it will become as much a part of the discipline of my living as resting and diets.

It is easy to write these words of good advice but very much more difficult to follow them. I know only too well how often I fail, get exhausted and feel unable to cope; but one must never give up hope. We only have one life on this earth and it often seems to me that it is going to take me rather longer than that to live sensibly with multiple sclerosis. One can only keep trying and perhaps on the way become a little more philosophical and a little more patient with oneself as much as with others, particularly those who are closest and dearest to us.

CHAPTER THIRTEEN

Multiple Sclerosis
and Work

Occupation is a vital part in keeping up morale during any illness and most particularly in a chronic and relapsing illness such as multiple sclerosis. It is more important for a man or for the main bread-winner to be able to carry on with gainful activity and not lose any sense of status or satisfaction in his life. Once again I think it is realistic, not pessimistic, to make an early assessment of the work that the person may be able to do at a later stage before a crisis occurs. Disablement and lack of mobility may occur very late but increasing fatigue is more likely to be an earlier problem. You may be able to carry on with your work with continuing and increasing fatigue but if at the same time you still want to enjoy life and your family it is better to face the fact that fatigue will very likely be a problem and it is better to make plans for the future earlier, rather than later.

If you can manage the job you had when multiple sclerosis was diagnosed it is so easy, especially if you have a good boss, just to go on in the same way ignoring fatigue and not thinking about the future. Perhaps for some people with especially strong ostrich tendencies this may be the best way, and for many people it may give them greater peace of mind and confidence about the future. It is very important that you should work as long as possible because it will keep you occupied, restore your morale and also increase your income. It does cost more to live if you are disabled and you are going to need all the money you can get in order to maintain a reasonable standard of living and enjoy a few extra pleasures like holidays and outings.

The Department of Employment can give you a great deal of advice about employment and I will talk more about this in Chapter Seventeen on statutory services for the disabled. Some of this information may be of great value to you but particularly if you already have a skilled training or profession, you may prefer to try and sort out your own future in your own way. I am going to talk mainly to such people in this chapter.

You may think as I did, that having recovered from an acute episode of multiple sclerosis you can go back to your old work, forget all about being ill and just carry on as before. Perhaps you will manage for a while and if you can I wish you joy but on the other hand you may find as I did that you cannot go on as before. I was fortunate because I was able to cut down my work commitment strictly to half-time which it had been theoretically before I was ill. I had, and still have, a marvellous boss who trusts me to get my work done and if I have bad days I make my work up on better days. I have nearly always managed to honour my fixed commitments although at times my family has suffered from my excessive fatigue through doing this particular work.

Even with my advantages at work and the privileges I enjoy, I am aware that the time is coming or sometimes seems to have come when I should be very much better and happier to be free to work when I felt most able to do so. There would be no fear of my becoming idle and restless because I am not like that. I do realise however, that if I stopped going out to work I should run the risk of hibernating and miss the stimulus of the company of the congenial people I meet while I am working. At the moment it is in the balance. I am aware of the advantages of not having to drag myself out to a fixed work commitment when I am too tired to manage it but on the other hand I still get great pleasure from meeting other people when I am out and doing my very varied work. Meantime I keep a foot in both worlds and gently increase my writing commitments with a less mobile future in mind. I have invested in a good tape-recording machine with a microphone and have found a secretary who can do audio typing. Perhaps this sounds pessimistic but typing has become increasingly arduous with weakening back muscles. Now I am content to wait and see how things develop and continue to potter along with medicine for the moment. During the good weeks I feel that I should be able to carry on working part-time away from home for another ten years or so but during the bad weeks I just long for the time when I shall be mistress of my own time and only have to move away from my home when I choose to.

I feel, and I think, many others with multiple sclerosis would agree with me that great ambition in any career has to be abandoned. Examinations cause stress and anxiety and both of these may produce relapses in multiple sclerosis. If you want to get to the top in any profession you have to work long hours and often under great physical and mental pressure. If multiple sclerosis is diagnosed early in your career I should say it is better to choose a good steady line in your profession rather than go for anything less certain, less secure and more demanding. For instance, it would probably be better to aim at a speciality with fewer emotional demands and not too much night work in the profession of medicine. Whichever medical speciality I suggested some doctor would feel slighted but I think many in the medical profession would agree that pathology would be a less demanding speciality than that of surgery. There would also be the possibility later of working less than a full number of sessions. Geriatrics is another possibility. It is always under-staffed and while working in an under-staffed speciality it is often easier to manage to do part-time work. I know that in dentistry it is possible for dentists in private practice and in the school dental service to do less than full-time work.

Possibly it is ideal to be self-employed if one has the ability and capital for such employment. Obviously the employment must not depend on the expenditure of too much energy unless the work is undertaken with friends or with a family. The administrative part of the work in a small factory, business or hotel could well be undertaken by a patient with multiple sclerosis. Accountancy is always a good and reliable profession. I have no first hand knowledge of practising part-time accountancy but I would think that it was a suitable profession for arranging one's own hours.

If you have any creative talents it is a good idea to have serious thoughts about developing them early in the illness. You may say it is quite pointless because you only daub and could not possibly paint, or that you love writing letters but could not write anything that would be published. I think there are two fallacies here. The first is that creative hobbies do not have to be looked on as potentially lucrative now or later. It is far more important for you as a person to develop something that is pleasurable for you and gives you a sense of achievement. It is so easy to feel downhearted that a degenerative disease is getting at you and I think one of the best antidotes to this sort of doldrum of the spirits is to create something so that not only the creation itself but also the pleasure in creation are rewards enough.

The second fallacy is that hobbies at which you feel only moderately competent could not possibly be sources of income now or later. This just is not true. If your hands are still nimble there is always the demand for simple dressmaking, knitting or alterations. You do not need professional training for much of this work; avoid tailoring work unless you have had the experience! So many people are terrified of doing the simplest alteration on a dress but they are quite prepared to pay you to do what for some people are simple things like turning up hems or putting in new zips. I know somebody who has become expert at creating, and creating is the word, lampshades for which she can justifiably charge a good price.

A breadwinner or a potential breadwinner for the family may want to make his/her own plans early in the illness and independently rather than seeking official government help. Some men and women will choose to go to part-time day or evening classes to learn a new skill such as secretarial work, some may wish to take a university degree either through the Open University or as an external student at a university. A friend of mine who is disabled, although not from multiple sclerosis, is a qualified chemist but was unable to continue with a full-time job. He has started a small but thriving perfume factory. The possibilities are endless but you must think about this early while you are mobile, more energetic and enterprising and while you are more able to see your hopes and ambitions materialise.

Journalism can be a useful and paying hobby. Freelance journalism can be quite lucrative but is unlikely to provide a good and steady income unless you are very fortunate. Full-time staff journalism is an energetic and physically and mentally exacting profession and not likely to be suitable for somebody with multiple sclerosis, certainly not later in the disease. If you feel like trying freelance journalism or short story writing, or writing plays for radio or television it can be a good idea to do a correspondence course to get you started. I have had some dealings with the London School of Journalism and found them reliable, responsible and constructive in their help. I know many people manage to get articles or stories into print without such help but for others, professional help and encouragement may be very necessary. Even if you never succeed at making money at writing it might be a very interesting hobby for the day when you may become less mobile. It is worth investing in a typewriter early in your efforts as a journalist because you will not be made welcome by any editor if you send him work that is hand-written. If it is financially possible an electric typewriter is a better investment for somebody with multiple sclerosis than an ordinary typewriter because far less effort is necessary to use the keys and this could be very advantageous if your fingers get weaker.

You will gain if you can live near your work because you will save much of the fatigue of travelling. Fatigue is certain to be inevitable and if you can possibly manage even half an hour lying down in the middle of the day it can be of great help. If you are unsteady walking either on your way to work or at work it is far better to use a stick than to keep stumbling. Possibly it also serves to remind you and your workmates of your limitations. I have to confess that I still suffer all the indignities of tripping over and bumping into things rather than make the decision to use a stick. It is probably a decision about as sensible and logical as a short-sighted adolescent who refuses to wear glasses. I have managed now to use a stick on rough roads and paths but leave it hidden at other times.

I think it is better to be honest with your workmates about your illness and about any disabilities you have. Having told them there is no need to belabour the point. I have found that frankness is repaid by kindness and understanding and if you are away from work for any reason to do with multiple sclerosis it is less likely to be considered that you are skiving from work. Most people are very willing to help if they know that help is necessary.

It is essential that your employer and your foreman, if you have one, should know that you have multiple sclerosis because it may be necessary to make some modifications to the tools you use or the position in which you work. If you are already disabled and in a wheelchair, access to the building may have to be made as well as suitable access to toilet facilities. These are already being made in newer buildings but may have to be installed in older ones.

CHAPTER FOURTEEN

Doctors

In the United Kingdom it is usual to have a general practitioner. There are very few people who do not have one even though they may seldom see him. If you have multiple sclerosis it is particularly important that you should have a general practitioner and it is even more important that you should have one whom you not only like and trust but in whom you have great confidence. However well you may feel at times, there are going to be other times when you will need medical advice, if not medicine, and it is as well that there is a medical presence however far in the background he remains for the majority of the time.

If you have not already got a doctor or if you have moved to a new area you will have to choose a doctor. A doctor or nurse is not allowed to recommend a doctor to you for ethical reasons. You can find a list of local practitioners at any post office and you are supposed to choose one off that list. If you live in a country area there may, in fact, be no choice of doctor which can make the matter simpler. If you live in a more densely populated area it may be wise to make a few discreet enquiries among friends and neighbours before deciding which doctor to choose. When you have made your choice take your medical card to the doctor of your choice and ask if you can register with him. If you register with a group practice you may not be able to state the doctor of your choice because patients will be allocated to each doctor according to the number of patients technically on his list. You are likely to be able to see the partner of your choice if you call at the surgery but there may be some zoning of doctors for home visits. The medical notes from your previous doctor may take a little while to reach your new doctor because they will have to go through several offices.

If you have lived in an area for many years before developing multiple sclerosis you may have been registered with the same doctor since before you were married and possibly had children. You may have found him very good about obstetrics and young children and there may have been few occasions when you have needed him yourself. It could be that, although you have known him for a long time and have no reason to doubt that he is a good doctor, the situation could change when you know that you have developed a chronic illness and there will be other qualities that you require in your medical adviser. You could reach a point where you are hesitating about a change of doctor, and will have to face the fact that your needs and inevitably the connected needs of your family must take priority over your doctor's feelings. There is a widespread misunderstanding that you have to inform a doctor that you wish to leave his list; certainly you can inform him if you wish to. You may want to thank him for all his past help and perhaps explain why you wish to change. I had to do this on one occasion because we were still registered with a doctor for whom I had worked, when I had my own small children. I knew a certain amount of children's medicine and he had the disconcerting habit of asking me what I thought about my own offsprings' illnesses. Eventually I managed to write to him and explain that I valued the fact that he could still treat me as a medical colleague but with my own children I was just a flappy mother and must have a doctor who would treat me as such! He accepted my explanation very well and we remained good friends.

As I have said, to change your general practitioner take your medical card to the doctor of your choice and ask him if he will accept you on his list, and the transfer then goes through the normal bureaucratic channels. A doctor has the right to refuse to take you on his list, but he does not do this unless his list is overcrowded. A doctor on whose list you are already can also ask that you should be removed from his list. This is an unusual procedure and a doctor usually only resorts to it when relations have become unbearably strained between him and his patient. If no other doctor in the area is willing to take the poor unwanted patient, the Family Practitioner Committee has to allocate the patient to a doctor chosen by the committee. This procedure does not often happen but it always causes a certain amount of unpleasantness.

If you are choosing a doctor, when you already know you have a chronic illness, and are unlikely to move house frequently you will want to consider the arrangement as a long term plan. You may not want to see him frequently and this will depend not only on the severity or the relapses of your illness but also partly on your own self-sufficiency and your needs for encouragement and support. We all need some support at all times and especially when we are ill but our domestic circumstances, our characters and to some extent our normal resilience will determine the amount of medical help for which we must ask.

We all need to find a doctor who is not only sufficiently able to spot new trends in our illness but also has sufficient understanding and patience to be able to listen to the occasional tale of woe and give constructive advice. Unfortunately high intelligence, good clinical judgement and deep human understanding are not necessarily combined in one doctor. It really is asking a lot in any man of any profession and doctors are only human! It is going to be very difficult to decide whether sound clinical judgement or deep human understanding are going to be of greater need to you and then to know whether you are spotting the right quality in the right man. It is difficult enough choosing a doctor even if you have considerable wide inside knowledge of the member of the profession. I have a fair knowledge of the clinical ability of doctors for or with whom I have worked and also of those that I have heard speaking at medical meetings. I naturally hear a lot more from other mothers about what a certain doctor does or says and I have to be particularly careful not to get involved in any gossip about doctors or give any of my personal opinions. I cannot know however what a particular doctor will be like in a personal crisis involving myself or my family until such a crisis occurs. I think that the one sort of doctor that I should always avoid is one who is highly intelligent, very well qualified but lacking in human understanding.

A general practitioner in the United Kingdom must be medically qualified. This means that he has either degrees or recognised diplomas and has done the necessary work and paid the fee to have his name included on the General Medical Register. The General Medical Council which keeps this register also has a disciplinary body to which doctors can be reported for inappropriate behaviour or negligent work. A doctor can be reported by an individual or summoned to appear before the court.

A general practitioner may have his basic qualifications or he may have higher degrees; an increasing number of general practitioners do now have higher qualifications because more of them are doing a three-year postgraduate course of vocational training which is likely to enable them to sit one or more higher degrees. A general practitioner may have the M.R.C.G.P. (Membership of the Royal College of General Practitioners), the M.R.C.P. (Membership of the Royal College of Physicians) which is a high academic degree in general medicine and might well be of particular use to you if you have multiple sclerosis. He may have the D.R.C.O.G. or M.R.C.O.G. (Diplomate or Membership of the Royal College of Obstetricians and Gynaecologists), the D.C.H. (Diploma in Child Health), and various others. He may have achieved these examinations along the way towards general practice or he may have wanted to specialise in another branch of medicine for which he required the qualifications but has ended up in general practice. Neither way means that he could not be a first class general practitioner.

I think one of the most important attributes that any doctor, general practitioner or specialist, can have is to be able to talk to you as a person rather than over your head as an 'impersonal patient'. Perhaps this is particularly true in an illness such as multiple sclerosis where a loss of, or change in identity can play so important a part in the mental effects of your illness. If your doctor by his treatment of you and the way in which he speaks to you can make you feel more and not less of a unique individual he will have done you a great healing service. It may be difficult for a doctor, particularly one who has always revelled in good health, to understand just how important this approach is. It is probably more difficult and even more important to make good contact with any patient with a chronic and disabling illness. The doctor by his attitude can increase or can minimise our own feelings about handicap. He can help you to feel that you are still very much a person and that life has meaning for you, or he can help accentuate the feeling of being less than a whole person and in some ways an outcast, unwanted and unloved.

Everybody knows that general practitioners are very hard worked and it will help your doctor a lot if you can use his services so that you take up as little as possible of his time. A visit to the surgery, if at all possible, will take up much less time than a visit from him to your home. Demands for a home visit are usually required before 10 a.m. and demands for late evening or night calls should never be made unless it is a real emergency. Most problems in multiple sclerosis are going to be of long-standing and although the moment will come when you feel you must get help, the more reasonable and considerate you are of your doctor's time the more considerate he will be of your problem and the more of his time he will be likely to find for you.

You may realise when you think about the problem on your mind that it may not even come within the doctor's powers to help. In multiple sclerosis blowing over in a high wind can be a real problem. There is nothing the doctor can give you to solve the problem but a good handrail down some outside steps might stop the problem very effectively. You do not need to ask your doctor about this but see your local Director of Social Work and ask for his help. It will usually be given very promptly and that will save you falling and also your doctor's time. There are a few simple ways in which you and your doctor may be able to get on well together. When you see your doctor there will probably be a number of problems you want to ask him but if you remember them rather than producing a 'shopping list' and working through it he will be better pleased. If your doctor gives you medicine to take, do take it in the dose he has prescribed, and if it does not agree with you let him know. If he gives you advice about diet or reducing weight or taking exercise try to take the advice and do as he says. He will find far more time and find it far more willingly for a patient whom he finds is co-operative than for one who never takes any notice of the advice he has given.

One of the most frequent complaints patients make about their doctors now is that they have no time to listen. 'As I sat down to try and tell my doctor something he reached for his prescription pad and started writing.' I am sure this must happen because I have heard it said so often. I can only suggest that you keep your demands for medical help to the minimum and the doctor's time may then be more generously forthcoming. I have never met the problem but when I do need help or advice it is always available and if I have not seen my general practitioner for a while he usually phones up to make sure all is well. Naturally such an arrangement will depend on the character of both the doctor and the patient and the variations will be infinite.

Other doctors are called consultants or specialists. These doctors have higher qualifications in their chosen speciality and will have spent at least ten years undergoing a gruelling hospital training after qualification. Not all of them will make it as far as consultant status but from those who do one can expect a very high standard of medical expertise. Formerly there were many consultants in general medicine but during recent years this has tended to change so that there are now specialists in the narrower specialities such as neurology, cardiology, rheumatology and other subjects. If you have multiple sclerosis and see a consultant you are most likely to see either a neurologist or a general physician. This will depend in part on where you live and partly on the particular interests of the general physician.

There is no absolute reason why you should see a specialist, although most general practitioners would consider it desirable to confirm the diagnosis. You may seek a second opinion but this may not always be possible on the National Health Service.

If you want to see a particular doctor it may be wiser to ask to see him privately. One always hopes that a problem of this sort can be resolved as amicably as possible.

Multiple sclerosis is an illness with a variable outcome and many spontaneous improvements and it naturally attracts quack remedies. If you are offered courses of injections or other forms of treatment, I think you would be wise to ask the advice of a competent neurologist before accepting any such offer. At best it would do no good and at worst it could do harm particularly to your bank balance.

CHAPTER FIFTEEN

Identity as Able
or Disabled

I do not think that I had ever seriously considered what disability could mean to a healthy adult until three years ago. Certainly I had had discussions with arthritic patients who were not all, but mostly older than myself. I had had very little to do with orthopaedic patients who had lost limbs. I was always surprised with what apparent facility people accepted mutilating hand surgery and afterwards made as useful an appendage of the hand as they could. I knew far more about the problems of patients with severe bronchitis or who had had colostomies. Both were disabled in the way in which they could live but somehow the word did not seem to be used very much.

I have known, and do know, very much more about handicapped children and their parents because I have done a lot of work with such families. About one per cent of all babies born have a major handicap but the enormous size of the problem is not fully realised because many of these babies do not live. A very great number of children have minor handicaps which range from birthmarks to an extra toe. A mother's first question after the delivery is nearly always, 'Is the baby all right?' Her second question is about the sex of the baby. I suppose this almost primitive insistence on the normality of the body and mind may stem from a time when only the fittest could survive. The very strong feelings of normality and abnormality or handicap are difficult to argue with or change because they are very deep rooted.

Having used the words abnormal, disabled and handicapped we are left wondering just what we mean. The grossly abnormal baby that is born with little or no brain or with a severe spina bifida or the absence of limbs obviously comes within the category of disabled. On the other hand the lack of a toe, although technically a disability, hardly comes within the same category. By the time a child reaches school age there are ten categories of handicap which may need special schooling. Many of these handicaps have not been observed at birth. The ten categories include the loss of hearing or partial hearing, loss of sight or partial sight, speech defects, physical and mental handicap and behaviour disturbances. You can see that in many of these conditions the distinction between variations of normal and handicap is narrow and in this instance handicap is only used as a description for purposes of education.

Disability is not going to be something that goes away, in fact it increases all the time. Medical advances may prevent the birth of some handicapped children such as mongols who can be detected early in pregnancy and an abortion can be carried out if the mother so wishes. On the other hand medical advances also save the lives of many babies born with severe handicaps who would previously have died. At present there is much discussion about the worth of doing expensive, serious and repeated operations on children whose life will always be very limited both physically and mentally. No doctor would say that such children should be deprived of life but only that they might have less suffering if not exposed to heroic surgery when there is very little hope of real enjoyment in life ever being attained.

Disability does not just apply to children who are born with handicaps, or to those who develop diseases such as multiple sclerosis, but to all those conditions that happen to so many of us in time even if we have had healthy lives. Many people will develop arthritis which can be extremely disabling; heart disease which restricts their activity considerably; or high blood pressure and strokes. The list is very long and as few people die at a younger age from diseases such as tuberculosis, more live to get the diseases associated with growing old. Therefore the number of handicapped people, both those growing older who have been born with a handicap and those who are living longer, are going to increase and the problem on a social and economic level is also bound to increase. In the United Kingdom there is now a Minister for the Disabled; a great deal of work has been done to help the disabled and many more plans are under way. This will be discussed more fully in Chapter Seventeen on statutory and Chapter Eighteen on voluntary services.

Here I want to talk more about the personal meaning of being able-bodied or disabled. A handicapped child, apart from the discomfort he may have to put up with, is probably unaware of the fact that he is in any way different from other children until the age of two or three when he begins to mix more with other children. By five years most children are acutely aware of any visible differences in themselves such as malformed arms or legs or severe birthmarks. Those who often seem least affected by other children are those who are mentally handicapped. Adults seem more likely to notice their differences than other children. Small children seem to have little difficulty in accepting other small children who are mongols.

As handicapped children go through school, some become acutely aware of being different and in a way apart from the usual run of children. This can happen to very intelligent children with severe physical abnormalities such as muscular dystrophy. They probably manage quite well in a wheelchair through primary school, where the building may well be on one level. Suddenly the time comes for secondary education and it is impossible in the great majority of normal secondary schools because there are too many stairs and no lifts. A school for the physically handicapped may be insufficiently academic. Sometimes the only solution is home tuition. This may be acceptable academically but can mean a very isolated life with few friends and interests outside the home.

These children certainly realise they are different by the time they come to get jobs. Although there are regulations about the employment of handicapped people there are so many opportunities closed to them. Even the very bright children find getting to university a real problem. It is no good going to university, however well qualified you are, if you are unable to get your wheelchair into a lavatory. Stirling University is a marvellous example of a university designed so that disabled students can be fully integrated into the community. There are the few grossly handicapped who have, against amazing odds, achieved a great deal. One thinks of Helen Keller, but the very fame of those who achieved much makes one more aware of the great number of disabled students who must be under-achieving.

I have talked about handicapped children and their growth in some detail because I think it has considerable bearing on our own reaction to personal disability when it is met much later in life. I think that the profound effect it has on the mind of most people is caused by the conditioning with which we have grown up. There are those people who are normal and able-bodied and there are those who are abnormal in some way and disabled. I might even add that the former is also considered essentially likeable and attractive, and the latter considered not to be liked and unattractive. To have had the pleasure of meeting and speaking to Dr. Margaret Blackwood is to see the latter belief blown sky-high. She is a Scottish woman, severely disabled with muscular dystrophy, who has spent her life fighting for the rights of the disabled, and for which she was made an Honorary Doctor of Law by Aberdeen University; she is now confined to a wheelchair and is very weak, but few people could be more radiant or attractive, wheelchair or no wheelchair. I think that there is a reason for this; she has achieved what should be the goal of every disabled person—to become a whole person in spite of a disability.

An adult's mental attitude to disability may be the reason why disability is frequently felt first in the mind before it is noticeable or possibly demonstrable in the body. I think there are very few people who realise this, including doctors. Perhaps if a doctor was told of this strong feeling of disability in a patient who showed either no or minimal signs of disability, he might be tempted to dismiss it as some form of neurosis. This distressing mental feeling of disability can be a strong force for possibly many years before there is any visible, or what might be called actual, disability. It is difficult either to produce figures on this or a large number of cases, and as I have said elsewhere sufficient evidence is necessary to show anything as a fact rather than just an idea or an opinion. I am not giving this as a fact but as a personal impression based on my own experiences and on several long discussions with those in a similar position who would not be labelled neurotic in a general sense. If disability is really an attitude of mind as much as a physical fact different methods are going to be needed in order to compensate anybody totally for disability. Perhaps compensation is the wrong word because nothing can put damaged myelin sheaths together the same way again and a damaged nervous system will remain damaged.

On the other hand it may be possible to aim at being a whole person again in spite of considerable physical and mental damage. Some multiple sclerosis sufferers appear content to put up with the pieces and even make their disabilities a major part of their conscious life. On lists of some members of voluntary societies a 'D' or an 'M.S.' goes against those who are disabled or known to have a disease. Sometimes quite surprisingly strong feelings can erupt that one of these classifications has been put against a name misguidedly. Perhaps she is not in a wheelchair and can get around with one elbow-crutch. I think it is only because a person who passes such judgement has come to accept a fragmented life, that she can feel so strongly about things, to which others seem very trivial. Anybody with a crutch is disabled in one sense but perhaps the person who objects to this interpretation is as much mentally disabled as physically disabled.

I do not know the answer to attaining wholeness again but sometimes I have glimpses of what it could mean. I feel certain that it has remarkably little to do with the degree of physical disability but to one's attitude to it. Doctor Margaret Black-wood as previously mentioned, speaks with her characteristic courage and enormous humour of the 'non-disabled' and perhaps that phrase really does mean something. A great deal has been achieved in the past five years in the United Kingdom, to make any sort of disability more respectable. A wheelchair sign indicates hotels which cater for people in wheelchairs. Tourist offices will give advice on restaurants and other public facilities which are accessible to wheelchairs. Legislation has made it necessary for all new public buildings to have toilet facilities for the handicapped. New allowances and pensions are being introduced with the prime aim that all people, disabled or non-disabled, have the right to an independent existence and that disabled people do not want to exist on charity or to be forgotten in the less noticed wards of older hospitals. All of these things are steps in the right direction but there are still enormous problems which have to be solved at a personal level. There are few people with the expertise or the experience to whom one can turn for guidance in these intensely personal and sometimes very difficult problems.

Perhaps living in a materialistic society creates its own problems. On the one hand disability can be faced superficially by keeping a trim figure, dressing well and bothering about hair and make-up. These all conform to the accepted values of the society. On a deeper level the opportunity for a good and possibly university level of education may help to detract from some of the socially felt stigmas of disability. A girl in a wheelchair who had a university degree was travelling with her fiancé. She was never asked a question about a passport or a form but the question was always referred to her able-bodied fiancé who was pushing the wheelchair. The attitude of stigma lingers on, and must rub off on to the newly disabled.

I think it is very important to keep in contact with good friends who, by their acceptance of you, are able to help you feel less of a non-person. You must be prepared to mix with people. Try to summon the courage to meet new people, by learning to take an interest in other people and their lives and interests and problems. I think it really does help to re-build you as a whole person. There will be many failures when you fall down in your endeavours and slip back into the feelings of being maimed and damaged and in some way broken.

For those who have a belief in a power greater than themselves, more help is available. I am not using the word Christianity exclusively because I think any of the great religions of this world has the power to make a person whole again. It may be impossible for many to believe in such a power, but for those who do, they may receive healing; a great restoring process can be achieved through the power of prayer, not only through their own prayer but through the prayer of friends and religious communities. In all the difficulties of each day it is all too easy for those who believe in this power to forget and lose hope—but that power is always there, waiting for the asking.

There is no simple answer to distinguishing between disabled and able-bodied and even less is there a simple answer to restoring disability, not only of the body but of the mental attitude to it. It is a way which I think we each have to find for ourselves, depending on our own character and background and beliefs. I am sure it can be done given sufficient time and hope and courage, but we shall all fall by the way, metaphorically speaking, many times. Then all we can do is pick the pieces up and keep on trying. Despair is the worst disability of all.

CHAPTER SIXTEEN

Sources of Information

opening quote.

When I was first told I had multiple sclerosis, I was inundated by remarks that it must be far worse for me because I knew all about it. Well, I knew surprisingly little about it even for a doctor. In fact I knew the absolute minimum that would get me through my examinations! The second thing that struck me was the fact that it must in some way be worse to know anything about a disease from which one is suffering. If that is so, it is surprising how often one hears a patient or his relatives complain that they were told nothing or practically nothing about the illness. I have never heard a complaint that anybody was told too much; only that they were told badly and with too little understanding.

The truth of what should be told or left untold must be different for every patient and even vary from time to time for the same patient. I said at the time the diagnosis was made, and I meant it, that I wanted to be told the truth so that I could understand what I should have to cope with. Now, I know that request was rather naïve and I am well aware that I should be quite glad to be told most of the truth, possibly even touched up a little. At times I find speech difficult, but I do not wish to think or be told what part of my anatomy is affected and what the eventual outcome is likely to be. I know already that it is much worse when I am tired and improves when I am rested and I am quite content to be told just that and encouraged with a little sincere and professional optimism. What an ostrich and what a hypocrite! I can say to the long-suffering neurologist, whom I see from time to time, that I want to be told everything and yet remain confident in his wonderful and possibly super-human understanding of just how much I really do want to know. It must be more constructive for my health to know that adequate rest will improve a symptom which is troublesome at the moment, than to know what might happen in another year or even in another five years time. I am fortunate that I trust my general practitioner and I trust the neurologist and if I want to ask a question I ask it and never suffer from doubts about the truthfulness of the answer I am given. Whether it is the whole truth I do not want to know, but I am sure that it is nothing but the truth.

Not everybody is as fortunate and we all know stories about patients who have been admitted to hospitals for investigation and have only discovered they have multiple sclerosis by over-hearing a conversation not meant for their ears or having a fur-tive and forbidden glance at their case notes. I wonder if these patients had already given the impression that they would get very upset if they were told the diagnosis. They will certainly get justifiably upset if they find out by subterfuge but perhaps they could have made it clear before, to a doctor in charge of them, that they really did want to know what was wrong with them and that they were going to behave quite responsibly when told. I know how difficult it is in hospital to get a quiet word with the doctor. His bleep keeps on going, or sister wants him or he just is not looking your way when you try to catch his eye. Communications in hospital leave a very great deal to be desired and it is not just a facetious joke that many patients can get more information from the ward maid than the doctor in charge of their case. It is a sorry state of affairs and one that should be remedied but so far no suitably effective way has been found in training young doctors in better methods of communi-cation. Various methods are being tried including interviews with actors which are then played back on video cassettes for discussion and criticism by a class of students.

At the moment, however, you are at the mercy of your doctor and it is up to you to let him know that you really do want to know the truth or as much of it as he thinks you want to know. You must also let him realise that you are not going to become hysterical or despondent when you are told. After you have been told the diagnosis and you have had time to think about it, there are going to be more questions that you will want to ask and other things you will want to know. It is a great help if you have a follow-up appointment with a neurologist because you may then have your questions answered. If you wish to check on the academic credentials of the specialist to whom you are referred, you can look him up in the British Medical Directory to be found in most public libraries. You can get a rough estimate of his age from his date of qualification at which time he would probably have been about twenty-three. He will have either an M.R.C.P. (Membership of the Royal College of Physicians), or F.R.C.P. (Fellowship of the Royal College of Physicians). If you look at his list of past and present jobs, many of them will be in neurological work and his published work will be also on neurological work. Look particularly for published work on multiple sclerosis.

It is obvious that no doctor, however well informed and however understanding, is going to be able to give you exactly the right amount of information at the time you most require it. Like small children wanting knowledge, ill people have times when they really do want answers and other times when they prefer to keep thoughts of illness out of their minds. An easily available source of information is the *Encyclopaedia Britannica* in the public library. You may be able to get ready access to nurses' textbooks; some of them are well written and informative but they do tend to write at length on the terminal nursing of multiple sclerosis which is necessary but not very encouraging for those who are still mobile and optimistic about the future.

It is usually more difficult to find medical textbooks to read and again I should advise you not to do it. They tend to stick to well established facts about illness, which is commendable but they are intended for students needing to pass examinations and not for the mental enlightenment of patients, even medical patients. I made a personal resolve that I would not look in a medical textbook after the diagnosis of multiple sclerosis was made. I kept that resolve until I came to write this book and I was more or less forced to look in a few textbooks in order to attempt to write the second chapter of this book! I was very glad indeed that I had kept my resolve previously because I do not think I could have avoided depression from the catalogue of possible complications and the various ways in which death may occur. I can only suppose that the budding physician does not need to acquaint himself with all the possible lines of treatment or even attitudes of mind which may bring hope and a greater drive to go on living each day. All I can conclude is that textbooks are definitely not suitable sources of information for multiple sclerosis patients unless they really want to revel in misery and pessimism.

Having downed orthodox medical textbooks as a source of information for patients with multiple sclerosis I must try and make some more positive suggestions. It is very difficult to find a book about multiple sclerosis that is reasonably in line with orthodox medical thinking and gives a balanced picture of what the disease can be. Most of the shorter and more readable books are either written by doctors with a very individual view of the disease or else by patients who give witness to remarkable personal recoveries. Both are interesting but I have found that I want a more balanced, well informed and less prejudiced view. One of the best balanced, most readable and thoroughly sensible articles about multiple sclerosis appeared in *Good Housekeeping* a few years ago, written by Wendy Cooper. I met it soon after I had been told I had multiple sclerosis and I found it gave me all the information I wanted. Much of it I must already have known, but conveniently forgotten, and the article was sufficiently encouraging and optimistic in outlook, to give me hope without allowing me to feel I was being hoodwinked. I read that article many times and I imagine it must have been of help to countless others like myself who were hoping for many active years ahead of them but who could not rule out the eventual possibility of immobility. I have been sent several articles from the popular women's magazines and also one or two from health magazines. I have found those from women's magazines overdramatic and, in many instances, inconsistent and inaccurate. Those from health magazines I have found interesting but they are all based on the individual experiences of one person who has taken up one particular diet or regime. I find these articles interesting but possibly it is my scientific training that makes it very hard to accept so biased an account without any commentary or professional control.

The weekly medical magazines can be a useful source of information. The *British Medical Journal* may be hard reading for all, including doctors. It is always worth reading the summary and discussion of the most abstruse article on multiple sclerosis if you can get access to the *British Medical Journal*. It can often be found in the public library. At least you are unlikely to be upset by such articles because your complaint is more likely to be inability to understand the distressing information! *Pulse*, *Doctor*, and *General Practitioner* at times have good articles on multiple sclerosis including up to date research and management. If you are able to borrow these from a medical friend they can be well worth reading. I find them encouraging rather than discouraging and often optimistic in outlook.

In 1974 there was a symposium on multiple sclerosis research sponsored by the Medical Research Council and the Multiple Sclerosis Society. It was held in London and neurologists with special expertise in multiple sclerosis from all over the world were present. The whole proceedings of the research were published in 1976 by Her Majesty's Stationery Office. The book is called *Multiple Sclerosis Research* and costs £5. Parts of it are difficult to understand but it is full of interesting ideas about multiple sclerosis and lines of research. The *British Medical Bulletin* of January 1977 is entirely devoted to multiple sclerosis. It costs £4.50 and is published by the British Council at 10 Spring Gardens, London. It is shorter and easier to read than the research proceedings published in 1976. I found it full of interesting information and it is complete enough to give you a balanced view of present medical thinking about multiple sclerosis. I think that reading any research literature is a good idea because it gives you a good all round knowledge about developments and helps you to keep an objective judgement about emotive claims for what are too often bogus remedies. Research literature may be difficult to read but I do not find it in the least depressing.

M.S. News which is published by the Multiple Sclerosis

Society has informative articles designed for the lay reader and also reviews of other books on multiple sclerosis. I am a regular reader of *M.S. News* and find it informative, encouraging and at times very entertaining. There are still a great number of depressing advertisements but I suppose these are necessary. To offset the effect of an inevitably crippling disease, the development of *CRACK* which is intended for young multiple sclerosis sufferers has an enormously stimulating effect on the production as a whole. I think it must be a sound source of information and encouragement to the 100,000 subscribers.

Books such as *Multiple Sclerosis* by Ritchie Russell are interesting largely for the case histories. It is fascinating to realise how many forms multiple sclerosis can take but fatigue almost always plays a prominent part in bringing on relapses; one can also wonder in view of its legion manifestations, just how many cases are undiagnosed in the United Kingdom.

CHAPTER SEVENTEEN

Statutory Services

There are many statutory services available for your use in the United Kingdom if you are ill or disabled but the problem may be to find them. It must be stressed that you are not accepting charity by taking allowances of money and other services if you are disabled; you or your husband have paid for them in your insurance stamps and your income tax. You are only accepting some of the advantages of living in a Welfare State.

The services described here will be restricted to those most likely to be necessary if you have multiple sclerosis. There is a useful booklet available from your Social Work Department on *Help for the Handicapped Person* and this gives a good summary of all the services available, although many of them are not applicable to you. I shall describe the services under those provided by the Health Authorities, the Social Work Department, the Social Services and those concerned with employment.

Everybody has the right to the services of a general practitioner and he is the normal front line in the team of medical care in the United Kingdom. He can get you the advice of a specialist either in a hospital as an inpatient or as an outpatient, or as a domiciliary visit in your own home. Domiciliary visits by specialists are not repeated but done once for a patient who needs further help and is not able or may not be willing to go to a hospital. This service is not very likely to be necessary in multiple sclerosis. If you need medical help urgently and your own doctor is not available you can ask either his deputy or failing that any other National Health Service doctor to call on you.

Your doctor may work directly with the district nurse and the health visitor. He may arrange for either or both of these people to call if you need nursing or other help. The services of these highly trained nurses are free to everybody who needs them. If you are in bed for any while at home the district nurse will be likely to call daily or twice a day to make you clean and comfortable and be certain that you do not develop any pressure sores.

The health visitor may be asked to call by your doctor. You may be able to discuss many of your worries with her including those about your family. She can suggest and arrange to supply various aids such as walking aids or a wheelchair. Her job is advice and counselling rather than ordinary nursing although she has trained to be a nurse before she specialised in health visiting. Either the doctor or one of the nurses can arrange for any medical supplies you may need, such as incontinence pads, a bedpan or a commode. There is a full chiropody service available on the National Health Service and it could be that if you are older or if your legs are stiff you would benefit from skilled treatment by a chiropodist.

You may at times need hospital treatment and this will be arranged after discussion between your own doctor and the doctor at the hospital. All hospital treatment as an inpatient or as an outpatient is free, although some of your benefits may be cut if you are in hospital for a long time. If you are not able to use a car or public transport when you go to hospital you should enquire from the hospital or your own doctor about having suitable transport arranged for you.

While you are in hospital a big attempt will be made at getting you rehabilitated so that you can once again lead a more or less independent existence at home. You are likely to have the help of a physiotherapist to help with movement and weak muscles, an occupational therapist to go through all the routines involved in daily life such as eating and dressing yourself. She will also help you both with hobbies and possibly with new skills for gainful occupation. You may see a social worker who will help you to sort out those problems that have made it difficult for you to stay at home. If you are in a long-stay hospital you may find that you can be employed in a sheltered workshop doing simple work for which you are paid a small wage.

When you leave hospital, convalescence may be arranged for you so that you can get as fit as possible before returning to tackle the problems you left behind you at home. After you have left hospital you will probably have a follow-up appointment as an outpatient. Your doctor may suggest that you should see a social worker from the Social Services, or in Scotland the Social Work Department, or if you ask for any advice or help from this Department, a social worker will almost certainly be sent to see you at home to assess your needs. Do not look on this as an unwelcome invasion of your privacy but as a very real way of helping you. She may spot things that would help you and of which you had not thought.

This Department has wide ranging powers to give varied help to anybody who is ill or disabled. The actual amount that can or will be done to help will vary from area to area depending on the budget allowed the Department and also on the policies of the local director. In some areas, including the one in which I live, a very great deal of help is given. Usually a social worker assesses the needs of the patient and of her family and then works in conjunction with the doctor in charge of the case.

This Department also has the power to provide many things from hot lunches to telephones but is limited by its finances at the time of writing. Home helps are provided but the number of hours help has been limited for financial considerations. A home help for a patient with multiple sclerosis going through a bad patch can be of enormous help and sometimes prevents a hospital admission. You pay some or all of the cost of a home help depending on your own financial position.

Meals on Wheels are organised by the Department and if you are unable to cook for yourself, a hot lunch will be brought to your house. In some areas there may be day centres for disabled people. Transport is provided to these centres and there are facilities for occupation, social activities, hairdressing and chiropody as well as a hot midday meal.

Some of these Departments provide full laundry facilities for a patient with advanced multiple sclerosis who may not have control over the passage of faeces and urine. The doctor will provide incontinence pads but the Department may have a door-to-door laundry service.

In some areas telephones will be installed for disabled people living alone. Sometimes the telephone engineers help in this service by giving their time to install such telephones and thus reducing the costs so that more people may benefit from this service. Other amenities may be provided in your home if you are in financial difficulties, such as radio, television or even a washing machine. Again these amenities will depend on local finances and policy in the face of a reduced budget. Occupational therapy may be provided at home or in a day centre if a therapist is available. Adaptations to houses such as the fitting of handrails on steps, the provision of ramps, the adaptation of a kitchen for use by somebody in a wheelchair and even the building of a downstairs bathroom or lavatory may all be undertaken by the Social Services or Social Work Department. The cost may be shared between you and the Department. In a few areas special housing is being provided for disabled people. If you are in doubt about your eligibility for any of these aids you must ask.

A social worker knows what voluntary help is available in the area where she works and she may be able to arrange for your shopping to be done, your fire to be lit and perhaps your garden dug for you. She may also be able to provide recreational facilities either at a day centre or sometimes just for outings. Some Social Services or Social Work Departments provide holidays or they may work with societies such as the M.S. Society. They may help with the cost of the holiday and the fares.

Adult training centres are provided which will give sheltered employment. Some centres are for all disabled people including those who are mentally handicapped. If you have been off work for a while but are hoping to get back, a training centre can be a useful half-way house where you will have to keep to regular hours but will earn a little money.

You may also get help in appealing against the rates on your house if you are disabled, getting help with the road tax on your car in certain circumstances and getting a disabled badge for your car. This badge helps you with parking near shops in areas where parking is normally forbidden.

If and when you are no longer able to live at home in spite of all aids the Social Work Department will help you find residential accommodation either in one of their homes or one run by a voluntary society such as a Cheshire Home.

The Social Security Department which is part of the Department of Health and Social Security will help with your finances. The allowances that are payable are constantly changing in number and amount but are always improving. I will give a brief outline of some of those available at the time of writing. You can get leaflets on all the allowances from the Department or from your local Post Office and if you want help somebody from the office will see you and advise you.

Ordinary sickness benefit will be paid for up to twenty-eight weeks if you are ill or disabled and have paid the necessary insurance contributions. Invalidity pension is paid after this time if you are still unable to work and to this invalidity allowance may be added. There is a non-contributory invalidity pension which in November 1977 was made available to married women for the first time as well as to others.

Other allowances for which you may be eligible if disabled are the mobility allowance, the attendance allowance which may be for night or day or both and the invalid care allowance for the person who stays at home to look after a disabled relative. Allowances that are paid to able-bodied people such as the maternity allowance will also be paid to you if you are disabled but in the same situation, for example pregnant.

The Department of Employment may be of help to you in various ways. You can be advised whether it will be of advantage to you to register as a disabled person. All firms employing over twenty people have to employ a certain percentage of registered disabled people. This may help you to get employment. If through disablement you are no longer able to do your former work you can have the advice and help of the Disablement Resettlement Officer (D.R.O.). He can arrange for you to have retraining if necessary at a special centre and will help you get suitable employment.

CHAPTER EIGHTEEN

The Voluntary Societies

The main voluntary society involved with multiple sclerosis is the Multiple Sclerosis Society or M.S.S. This society was founded in the United Kingdom in 1953 because of concern about the large numbers of sufferers from the disease. It is affiliated to over twenty other M.S. Societies throughout the world and through them to the World Health Organisation. The head office of the M.S.S. in the United Kingdom is at 4 Tachbrook Street in London, and there are about 300 local branches scattered throughout the country. If you have not got one near you and would be interested in starting a branch you can contact the head office about the way in which to go about it.

Since its inception the main aims of the society have been twofold and both aims depend on raising money. The first aim has been medical research and well over £1,000,000 has been given to this end. A team of medical assessors decide which types of research should be supported. Sometimes the society sponsors research alone and at other times in conjunction with such bodies as the Medical Research Council. The money given may be used to pay the salaries of medical or other workers or for the purchase of pieces of equipment, some of which are for very specialised blood tests, and which can be very costly indeed.

The second aim of the society is to help individual sufferers from the disease in a variety of ways. The help may vary from counselling to socials or holidays. There are welfare officers at the head office in London who are not only trained nurses and health visitors but who have also had a special training in the problems connected with multiple sclerosis. This counselling service is available 24 hours a day. Some of the other branches have their own welfare officers who may not be as highly trained but who are nevertheless available to help patients with some of their many problems and to give comfort and support.

A further function of the society which has developed since its inception is the spreading of news. Every member of the society receives a quarterly copy of the *M.S. News*. Although there are an estimated 50,000 cases of multiple sclerosis in the United Kingdom this publication has the amazing circulation of 100,000 copies per issue and it is obvious that a great number of relatives and friends and others interested must be reading it.

During the past few years there has been a new development in the magazine called *CRACK* which is specially designed for the younger patient with multiple sclerosis. There are always research reports, often interesting book reviews, constructive articles and some very stimulating correspondence. I find myself reading the magazine with interest and I particularly enjoy the research reports and book reviews. Other publications by the M.S.S. include a monthly bulletin and advice sheets on a number of subjects including books, holidays, legal aid and hobbies.

The local branches of the M.S. Society hold regular meetings for their members. I was invited to go to one about three months after I had been diagnosed as having the disease. As with any other organisation which exists for the help of people with a particular disease it is impossible to give advice as to whether any particular patient should or should not attend the meetings. It must be a personal decision. I was very doubtful about going to that first meeting but looking back one particular incident occurred that was, for me, very constructive and helped to change my own attitude to having multiple sclerosis.

At that meeting I was introduced to another woman who is a wife, mother and who has had a professional training. We only spoke briefly but that contact has since become of great value to me. We do not see each other very often or talk a great deal but we have much in common and in a scattered community it is a great comfort and pleasure to know that a congenial and understanding friend is around. It was probably on account of this introduction that I continued to go to meetings and became a committee member.

I think, in order to keep a true perspective on the disease of multiple sclerosis and particularly since nearly half the sufferers from the disease are able to lead normal or near normal lives, it is important that those patients who are in remission or who have benign multiple sclerosis, should think about joining the society as well as those who are severely disabled. In this way it could be easier to break down barriers between the able-bodied and the disabled and the helper and the helped. If you attend meetings while you are active and feel able to help others, you may at another phase in the disease feel less resentment at receiving help rather than giving help.

I know that some general practitioners dissuade their patients from joining the M.S. Society with such remarks as 'it is not for people like you'. The doctor may prefer to forget about the multiple sclerosis especially if the patient happens to be a friend. Nevertheless the patient is both a patient and a person and may have needs and worries which she might find very difficult to discuss with her general practitioner. I am not suggesting that meetings of the M.S. Society are for discussion of 'My' symptoms or 'Your' symptoms. They are usually very much more constructive than that. Yet in *M.S. News* and in the branch meetings problems may be solved which it would be quite impossible for other people, such as healthy doctors, to understand.

In this way the M.S. Society can take a place in the growing number of self-help societies in addition to its existing commitments. Apart from self-help there is also the 24 hour telephone service available in London through which more expert advice can be gained.

The M.S. Society through its helpers and the money that it raises provides many other types of help for patients with multiple sclerosis. It runs holiday homes where patients can go with their families, not only for a holiday but for general rehabilitation. Sometimes a local branch will subsidise a holiday in a suitable place other than one run by the M.S. Society or help with the holiday by providing the money for the fares. The M.S. Society can pay for a telephone to be installed, pay for additions to houses, television sets, washing machines and new wheelchairs. Many of these could be provided by the Social Services or Social Work Department and sometimes it seems to me a pity to take money from the funds of a voluntary society to provide things which could and should be provided by a State Department. The Social Services or Work Department or any other local authority department is not empowered to give money for multiple sclerosis research but in many areas can and will install a telephone or provide a washing machine. Of course, if the amenity is not forthcoming that is different and financial help should be made available. Holidays of a specialised nature are also rather a different matter and I feel that the M.S. Society has a unique service to offer in this direction.

Every now and again the M.S. Society comes in for some adverse criticism about its religious trends and emphasis. Apart from the occasional formal service, I have not been particularly aware of this tendency myself. I think that any body of people concerned with a chronic and incurable illness may have their active or latent religious feelings heightened. For some people this may be anathema but for others a religious faith is a great help and should not be belittled. It may keep alive their hope, their faith in life and in a future, and give them courage, endurance and optimism when they most need it. However, it would, I feel sure, be wrong if an attempt were made to foist religious beliefs on to those who have none. I am equally sure that it is wrong to belittle or in any way undermine the faith of both the disabled and the able-bodied in the M.S. Society where these are held with conviction.

The British Red Cross Society and the St. John Ambulance Brigade are not primarily involved with multiple sclerosis but both can be of great help in the loan of wheelchairs, bedpans, bed rests, bed tables and other nursing appliances for use at home. These loans are made on a temporary basis until equipment can be provided through official sources or to tide a family over a temporary setback in a patient's condition. A relative of somebody who is severely disabled with multiple sclerosis would be well advised to take a course in home nursing with either the British Red Cross Society or the St. John

Ambulance Brigade. These courses are free, open to the general public and are usually run each year. The course is usually for two hours one night a week for six to eight weeks. During the course basic nursing skills are learned such as bed-making, use of a bedpan, lifting and avoiding of pressure sores. If you are unable to attend a course the joint manual in home nursing published by the two bodies is full of clearly written and illustrated instruction.

The Disablement Income Group (D.I.G.) is an action group representing all those disabled from whatever cause. D.I.G. believes that there should be a national disability income no matter what the cause of the disability or marital or insurance status of the patient. This pension would be designed to consist of two parts; one should be an expenses factor and the other a maintenance one depending on the income that the sufferer would have earned were he or she able to work. It is costly to be disabled in so many obvious and more subtle ways. Home help may be necessary beyond that available through statutory sources. More heating will be required for someone who has to remain inactive all day. Tradesmen often have to be employed to do jobs which for the able-bodied would be do-it-yourself matters. It is likely that any necessary hair dressing or dentistry must be done at the patient's home and at her expense. The mobility allowance is very unlikely to cover the extra cost of transport. Sometimes the only way that a severely disabled patient can survive is by going into a hospital for the chronically sick. D.I.G. believes that all people prefer to remain independent and do not wish to rely on charity. Besides fighting for material benefits, which have included the mobility allowance, and the non-contributory invalidity pension for married women, D.I.G. has done a great deal towards making disability more respectable and admissible in the community. It has campaigned vigorously for such basic rights as special access for wheelchairs to public buildings including Post Offices and libraries and the building of toilets designed for the disabled. Local branches have varying amounts of money and the greater part of this is sent to the headquarters in London and Edinburgh to finance the national fight for a better deal for the disabled.

The Voluntary Societies

In a disease where depression can play a very prominent part at times the Samaritans must be mentioned. They are an organisation of trained voluntary workers who can be phoned at any time of the day or night when you are feeling very low. The telephone number can be found in the local telephone directory or local paper. The Samaritan on duty will listen to your problem and arrange a personal interview if it seems necessary. The Samaritans are trained to a certain point and they always have the back-up services of a psychiatrist. At any time during any period of depression it is worth remembering the Samaritans.

CHAPTER NINETEEN

Facing the Future

I think that facing the future in a disease such as multiple sclerosis is best done a day at a time—or in the words of Alcoholics Anonymous 'just for today'. I have talked about making plans for a more distant future and I think this is necessary, but having done your planning for various contingencies and worked out a way of living which seems best for you it is right to learn to live one day at a time and let the present merge into the future imperceptibly.

I know that various changes have occurred to me apart from neurological ones. I know that I am more sensitive; I have lost some sort of physical and mental self-confidence which makes me more easily affected by upsetting situations or even conversations. I am very much more likely to be upset if I am already tired. If I mislay a valued possession I feel quite panic stricken until it is found. I am more upset by actual or even imagined criticisms particularly from those close to me. Perhaps I am more emotionally dependent on them than I was before but I think, with time, this is passing. Although I am more vulnerable in certain ways I am also very much more ruthless in other ways in taking decisions which involve my family or myself. I have decided my priorities and having done that I can take decisions with a clear mind and very seldom with any later regrets. I have certainly been responsible for hurting other people's feelings in taking some of these decisions but I have not made the decisions with any intention of hurt to others and I am thankful that these incidental hurts seem to heal well.

My own experiences have given me a greater insight and understanding in my medical work. Without mentioning myself or my health I am able sometimes to make contact more easily and understand the problems more profoundly. It is not always possible to give constructive help and advice but I hope that it is sometimes.

I am, or possibly I should say my children are, at risk because of an increased interest and involvement on my part. Again, I think this increased interest in the next generation is one way of adjusting to the vulnerability in my own life and future. When I am aware of this tendency in myself I try to put it right and possibly over-compensate by almost pushing my young into independence. Normally I should be concerned but now I am frequently over-concerned although I hope that for most of the time I cover up my involvement fairly successfully. Probably the young, do in fact, understand and we may be able to laugh about it together later when interviews, driving tests and other crises are all over. All families have their fraught times!

Possibly the same feelings of a vulnerable future have encouraged me to spend time on hobbies which have a sense of permanence about them. Tapestry is one of these and all the work is tramé so that it not only looks better but will last longer. I have mounted one finished tapestry on a round Victorian piano stool; another long Queen Anne tapestry foot stool has been mounted temporarily by a local craftsman until the real thing and the money to buy it is available. I have even gone as far as making tapestry samplers for my as yet unthought of grandchildren! As my younger daughter said, 'What on earth do you think you are going to do with all that junk?' but my older daughter and son have made it quite clear that they will be delighted to give homes to Mum's creations one day!

I have found that a sense of humour is a great asset. Every now and again I swing the driver's door of my Beetle shut with my left hand and find myself spread-eagled over the bonnet! This happens when I have forgotten to plant my feet firmly on the ground and has become a recurrent indignity. Perhaps it seems particularly absurd because it is a bright yellow Beetle and I am invariably watched in my curious attitude by my delighted Scottie as well as any other passer-by. It is far better to see a situation as ridiculous than upsetting or embarrassing.

I am learning to live at peace with the knowledge of a vulnerable future without optimism except for one thing, or pessimism. I am very much more able to be tolerant of any physical weakness in myself. Before 1976 I would never stop working because I had a cold but now I can allow myself the luxury of a day in the warm if I am not well. If I am tired I can go to bed really early with an easy conscience and not feel bound to beat another two hours activity out of myself as I should once have done.

More than ever before, I enjoy the day in hand with its work and contacts with family and friends. I get more conscious enjoyment out of sights that previously I might have taken for granted; the breakers over the lighthouse in a southerly gale, the full moon reflected in the sea, the whiteness of the snow-covered hills, the myriad lights of a modern fishing boat coming slowly into harbour in the deep darkness; or on a more prosaic level I revel in lively discussions and arguments with my family or a really good meal. Even without the animal fat I can still enjoy grilled steak and good red wine!

Perhaps the one thing that makes me break my resolution to keep my hoping for today is the possibility that my husband may retire in a few months time. After the strain and difficulties, the thought of being able to learn to live together again more successfully makes me absurdly glad. I hope that I shall have the patience to help him adjust to the difference in his life and the strength of mind to forget the problems of the past years. It could make so much difference to have another adult and a second parent around. There will be problems adapting but at least there will be the opportunity given to us to build a new future together—albeit a very different one.

I met a wonderful old lady the other day. She is eighty-two but I am not sure that she should be described as 'old'. She is radiant with health, beautiful, tranquil and full of life. She had just lost her bed-sitting room in London: 'I told the Chap up there,' (pointing skywards) 'in whom I have great faith that He had better do something about it. I could not find myself another bed and if He could not find one here perhaps He could up there because it was about time. But He found me one here by the afternoon.' So she goes on living alone cheerfully working for an advanced poetry speaking examination. She has real courage. She has learned to live each day as it comes to the best of her ability and has no fear for the future. With such courage and hope and trust all things are possible and in the end, repose is not failure.

Useful Books

ABC of Services and Information. The Disablement Income Group, 28 Commercial Street, London E1 6LR.

The British Medical Bulletin, January 1977. Published by the British Council, 10 Spring Gardens, London SW1A 2BN.

A Guide to British Rail—a Handbook for the Disabled. Available from the Royal Association for Disability and Rehabilitation, 25 Mortimer Street, London W1N 8AB.

British Rail and Disabled Travellers. Published by the Joint Committee on Mobility for the Disabled, Wanborough Manor, Wanborough, Guildford, Surrey GU3 2JR.

Coping with Disablement. Published by the Consumers Association, 14 Buckingham St., London WC2N 6DS.

Disability Rights Handbook. This is published each year.

Handicapped at Home, by Sydney Foott. Published by the Disabled Living Foundation and the Design Council.

Multiple Sclerosis—Control of the Disease, by W. Ritchie Russell. Pergamon Press.

The Multiple Sclerosis Diet Book: a Low-Fat Diet for the Treatment of Multiple Sclerosis, Heart and Stroke, by Roy L. Swank and Mary-Helen Pullen. Published by Doubleday and Co. Inc., New York.

Multiple Sclerosis Research. Published by H.M.S.O. in 1976.

M.S. News. This magazine is published quarterly by the Multiple Sclerosis Society.

Useful Addresses

Action for Research into Multiple Sclerosis (A.R.M.S.). 71 Grays Inn Road, London WCIX 8TR. They have a London-based counselling service 01–568 2255.

Age Concern, Bernard Sunley House, 60 Pitcairn Road, Mitcham, Surrey.

The British Red Cross Society, 9 Grosvenor Crescent, London SW1X 7EJ.

The Disability Alliance, 5 Netherhall Gardens, London NW3 5RN.

The Disabled Living Foundation, 346 Kensington High Street, London W14 8NS.

Disablement Income Group (D.I.G.), Attlee House, Toynbee Hall, 28 Commercial Street, London E1 6LR.

The Multiple Sclerosis Society, 4 Tachbrook Street, London SW1V 1SJ.

St. John Ambulance Brigade, 1 Grosvenor Crescent, London SW1X 7EF.

Department of Health and Social Security: see telephone directory for your local office.

Department of Social Services/Department of Social Work: see telephone directory for your local office.

Department of Employment: see telephone directory for your local office.

Samaritans: see telephone directory or your local paper.

Useful Information Relating to the U.S.A.

National Multiple Sclerosis Society Headquarters
205 East 42nd Street
New York
New York 10017

There are 158 Chapters of this Society and divisional addresses and telephone numbers will usually be found in the Yellow Pages Directory.

A SELECTED LIST OF USEFUL BOOKS

MS and Us. Barbara Beach. Exposition Press, Hicksville, New York.

Multiple Sclerosis and How I Live with It. Ray Bjork, M.D. Obtainable from Helena Letter Shop, 11 Placer, P.O. Box 489, Helena, Montana 59601.

Run from the Pale Pony: Coping with Chronic Illness. Ronald and Myra Sue Pruet. Baker Book House, Grand Rapids, Michigan.

Survive or Succumb. Marian Spector. Booklet produced by Jefferson Printing Co, St. Louis, Montana. (This is a book on practical hints for living with MS.)

The Helping Hand Self Help Devices. Edward Lowman and Howard Rusk. Institute of Physical Medicine and Rehabilitation and the Arthritis Self Help Device Office. New York University Medical Centre, New York.

The National Multiple Sclerosis Society is able to give a fuller list of available books and other useful information.

Index

A.C.T.H., 22, 23, 49, 50
Adult Training Centres, 124
Allowances, 125

Benign multiple sclerosis, 15
Bereavement, 33–7
Bladder, 21
Body image, 34, 35
British Medical Directory, 117
British Red Cross Society, 129

Cerebrospinal fluid, 19, 22
Clumsiness, 13, 21
CRACK, 120, 127

Department of Employment, 125
Depression, 22, 91, 92, 131
Diagnosis, 12, 15, 20
Diet, 16, 23, 34, 53–61
Disability, 110–4
Disabled students, 110, 111
Disablement Income Group, 130
Disablement Resettlement Officer (D.R.O.), 83, 125
District nurse, 121, 122
Double blind trials, 54, 55

Emotional upsets, 90, 93
Exercise, 62, 65
Euphoria, 21, 91

Family reactions, 86–8
Fatigue, 7, 8, 9, 13, 22, 28
Fats, 17, 57
Friends, 69, 74

General practitioners, 101–7
Geographical distribution, 16, 17
Giddiness, 21
Gluten, 23, 53, 54

Handicap, 108, 109
Health visitor, 122
Heredity, 18
Holidays, 128, 129
Home helps, 123
Home nursing courses, 129, 130

Immunisations, 37
Immunity, 17, 18

Journalism, 99

Labour saving gadgets, 46
Letters, 71–3
Linoleic acid, 23, 60
Lumbar puncture, 11, 12, 22

Malaria, 10
Marital problems, 83–5
Measles, 17
Medical textbooks, 117, 118

M.S. News, 119, 120, 127
Multiple Sclerosis Society (M.S. Society), 41, 120, 126–9
Muscle spasm, 21, 51, 67
Muscular dystrophy, 110
Myelin, 19
Myths, 25, 28, 30

Nerve, 19
Neurologists, 30, 115
Non-animal fat diet, 56–8

Occupation, 42, 43, 83, 95
Open University, 98
Optic nerve, 20

Pain, 21
Pernicious anaemia, 22
Physiotherapy, 23, 47, 66
Pregnancy, 8, 18
Psychiatric illness, 27, 28

Reading, 43
Remission, 16, 31, 55
Research literature, 119
Rest, 23, 47, 48, 62–4

Samaritans, 131
Sensation, 21

Signs, 15, 16, 19, 21
Social workers, 121, 123
Specialists, 106
Speech, 21, 115
Sprouting seeds, 59
Steroids, 19, 22
St. John Ambulance Brigade, 129
Stress, 97
Sunflower seed oil, 23, 58, 60
Symptoms, 15, 16, 21, 49

Telephone, 72, 73
Telling the truth, 29
Twitching, 21, 67

Valium, 51
Virus, 16, 17
Vision, 8, 20
Visual Evoked Response (V.E.R.), 22
Vitamin B$_{12}$, 51
Vitamin tablets, 59
Vomiting, 21

Weakness, 9, 20

Yoga, 65
Yoghurt, 58